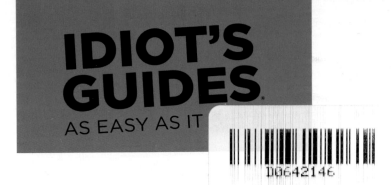

IDIOT'S GUIDES.
AS EASY AS IT

D0642146

High-Intensity Interval Training

by Sean Bartram

ALPHA

A member of Penguin Random House LLC

ALPHA BOOKS

Published by Penguin Random House LLC

Penguin Random House LLC, 375 Hudson Street, New York, New York 10014, USA • Penguin Random House LLC (Canada), 90 Eglinton Avenue East, Suite 700, Toronto, Ontario M4P 2Y3, Canada (a division of Pearson Penguin Canada Inc.) • Penguin Books Ltd., 80 Strand, London WC2R 0RL, England • Penguin Ireland, 25 St. Stephen's Green, Dublin 2, Ireland (a division of Penguin Books Ltd.) • Penguin Random House LLC (Australia), 250 Camberwell Road, Camberwell, Victoria 3124, Australia (a division of Pearson Australia Group Pty. Ltd.) • Penguin Books India Pvt. Ltd., 11 Community Centre, Panchsheel Park, New Delhi—110 017, India • Penguin Random House LLC (NZ), 67 Apollo Drive, Rosedale, North Shore, Auckland 1311, New Zealand (a division of Pearson New Zealand Ltd.) • Penguin Books (South Africa) (Pty.) Ltd., 24 Sturdee Avenue, Rosebank, Johannesburg 2196, South Africa • Penguin Books Ltd., Registered Offices: 80 Strand, London WC2R 0RL, England

International Standard Book Number: 978-1-61564-747-7
Library of Congress Catalog Card Number: 2014959611

17   16   15   8   7   6   5   4   3   2   1

Interpretation of the printing code: The rightmost number of the first series of numbers is the year of the book's printing; the rightmost number of the second series of numbers is the number of the book's printing. For example, a printing code of 15-1 shows that the first printing occurred in 2015.

Printed in China

Note: This publication contains the opinions and ideas of its author. It is intended to provide helpful and informative material on the subject matter covered. It is sold with the understanding that the author and publisher are not engaged in rendering professional services in the book. If the reader requires personal assistance or advice, a competent professional should be consulted. The author and publisher specifically disclaim any responsibility for any liability, loss, or risk, personal or otherwise, which is incurred as a consequence, directly or indirectly, of the use and application of any of the contents of this book.

Most Alpha books are available at special quantity discounts for bulk purchases for sales promotions, premiums, fund-raising, or educational use. Special books, or book excerpts, can also be created to fit specific needs. For details, write: Special Markets, Alpha Books, 375 Hudson Street, New York, NY 10014.

Trademarks: All terms mentioned in this book that are known to be or are suspected of being trademarks or service marks have been appropriately capitalized. Alpha Books and Penguin Random House LLC cannot attest to the accuracy of this information. Use of a term in this book should not be regarded as affecting the validity of any trademark or service mark.

Publisher: Mike Sanders
Associate Publisher: Billy Fields
Senior Acquisitions Editor: Brook Farling
Development Editor: Ann Barton
Design Supervisor: William Thomas

Photography: Matt Bowen Photography
Senior Production Editor: Janette Lynn
Indexer: Johnna VanHoose Dinse
Layout: Ayanna Lacey
Proofreader: Laura Caddell

For Rochelle—I want to make you smile for the rest of your life.

For Chloe—I am so incredibly proud of you. If I could give you one gift, it would be the ability to see you through my eyes. Only then would you realize how incredibly special you are and how much you are loved.

For Mum and Dad—as a parent I now know how hard it must have been to say goodbye, but despite the distance, I have never felt closer to you both.

"I can do all things through Christ who strengthens me."

—Philippians 4:13

CONTENTS

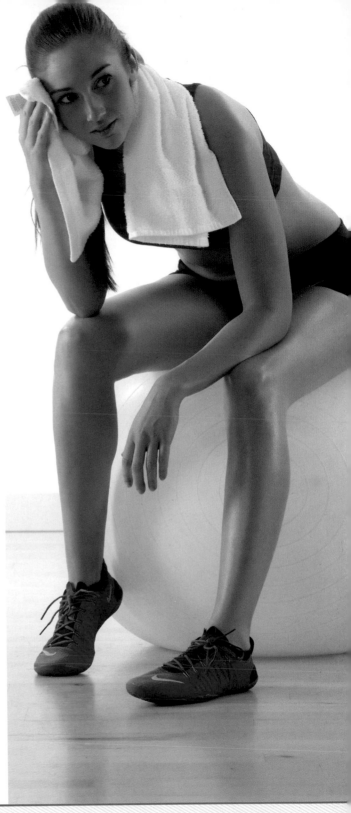

INTRODUCTION

If you picked up this book, then you've likely heard or read something about high-intensity interval training, or HIIT. Maybe you've heard that HIIT is a great way to get in shape without spending time and money at the gym. Maybe you've been logging hours on the treadmill and aren't seeing the results you want. Or maybe you'd like to lose weight for a vacation or special occasion.

Whatever your motivation, you're ready to begin. This book will guide you through your HIIT journey with 100 high-intensity routines differentiated by ability level, step-by-step instruction for 60 HIIT exercises, and tips and advice for nutrition, recovery, and monitoring your progress.

Get ready to work harder than you've ever worked before, because HIIT is all about maximizing your time and effort. It requires you to work at the height of your ability—but only for a short period of time. The key to HIIT is alternating short bursts of all-out intensity with short periods of rest. Studies suggest that this method of interval training is far more effective for burning body fat and increasing endurance than steady-state exercise, like jogging or biking.

PUSH YOURSELF

HIIT can be incredibly effective, but only if you work for it. If you only give 50 percent of the effort required, you can only expect 50 percent of the result. The key to HIIT is truly pushing yourself to the limit during the high-intensity intervals.

When you're training at a high level of intensity, you may feel uncomfortable, sore, and tired. You may even fail to finish. I encourage you to persevere. Giving it your all, even when uncomfortable, is the only way to have success!

In my studio I work with clients of all shapes, sizes, and ability levels. I've had motivated clients who have come in with significant weight loss goals and have achieved them thanks to these routines. We also have professional athletes who come in with incredible fitness levels and need to keep their bodies in top form. That's the beauty of HIIT; it can work for just about anyone. While most people undertake HIIT to lose body fat and shed a few pounds, it's equally effective for improving athletic performance, coordination, and core stability—essential tools to any athlete. No matter your ability level, starting point, or goal, if you are motivated and ready to put in a little sweat equity, HIIT will take your fitness to another level.

This book is designed to make your HIIT experience as easy as possible with exercises, workouts, and multi-day challenges that can be tailored to your schedule and your goals. Turn the page to learn more about HIIT and enter the exciting world of X-jacks, burpees, and skater jumps. It will be physically and mentally tough, but remember: good things come to those who sweat!

ACKNOWLEDGMENTS

Credit is due to so many incredible people who have contributed their time, energy, and talent to the production of this book.

Thank you to Alpha Books and DK Publishing for their faith in me and for making this project possible. A very special thank you to the "Dream Team"—my editors, Brook Farling and Ann Barton; our model, Breanna Fonner; and our photographer, Matt Bowen. Your enthusiasm and passion line every page of this book and it would not have been possible without each of you. I am very proud of all we have accomplished together and hope you are, too.

A huge thank you to my clients—your sweat provided the motivation for each page, and your dedication and commitment are my daily inspiration.

Sometimes the words "thank you" don't seem like enough for the people who have supported and believed in me. I may never be able to repay what these people have contributed, mentally, spiritually, and emotionally. To Clint and Gayle Bucher, Amy and Ben Breeze, Jess and Chad Frye, Jamie and Angie Volpert, the Zupancics, Erin Bell, Nicole Pollard, Kelly Tilley, and the incredible women of the Indianapolis Colts Cheerleaders—I shall forever be grateful.

The biggest thank you of all goes to you, the reader. I hope that this book challenges and inspires you, no matter what your end goal.

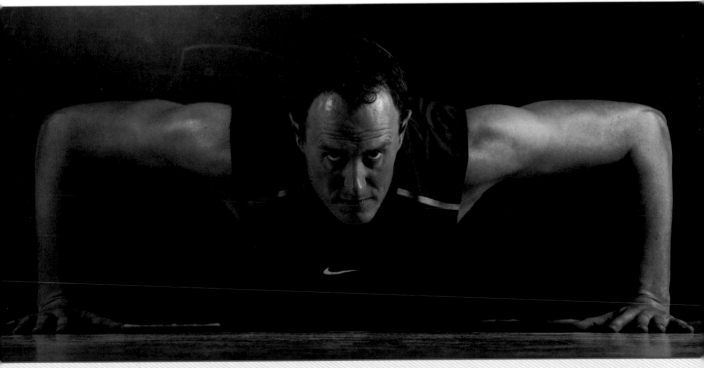

USING THIS BOOK

As with any exercise program, HIIT is not without risk. I strongly recommend that you consult a physician or primary health-care provider before undertaking this or any exercise program.

The use of this book is determined by your end goal. If weight loss, fat burning, increased muscle tone, and definition are your goal, the routines in this book will help you meet it. If you're looking to supplement your existing workout regimen, increase your athletic performance, or are simply intrigued by HIIT, you'll find inspiration and learn some new exercises to add to your arsenal.

COMPLETE THE FITNESS ASSESSMENT

The first step in your HIIT journey is to complete the fitness assessment. This simple tool is comprised of four foundational exercises. Your performance on these exercises will give you a baseline starting point, so you know the level at which you should be working out. The fitness assessment is not intended to recommend a particular course of action regarding your health, but it is meant to give you a sense of your current fitness level and provide a basis for you to create your fitness goals.

Once you've committed to a workout regimen, reassess your fitness every couple of weeks to track your progress and up the intensity if necessary.

CHOOSE A ROUTINE

So, you've assessed your fitness and you know where to begin. The next step is to choose a routine. The routines in this book are organized by difficulty.

Level 1 If you're new to HIIT or just getting back into working out after a long hiatus, this level is for you.

Level 2 This is the intermediate level. It's best for those who work out relatively regularly but aren't quite ready for the intensity of Level 3.

Level 3 This level is for those who are in shape and looking for a challenge.

You don't need to do the routines in order (although you can). Pick one that looks fun and challenging and fits your schedule.

READ THE ROUTINE

Before beginning a routine, review the exercises and make sure you know how to perform each one. If you need guidance, check the exercise section for instructions and practice a few times.

The routines range in length from a few minutes to nearly an hour. The "Total Time" includes repetitions and rest times.

During the "Work" intervals, you should do as many reps of the exercise as possible. Push yourself hard and keep moving until the interval ends. During the "Rest" intervals, you can stop moving and catch your breath or take a sip of water. As soon as the "Rest" interval is over, start the next exercise.

Some routines switch from one exercise to another without a break. If the rest time is —, go on to the next exercise as seamlessly as possible, without resting.

The routines are organized into sets and rounds. A *set* is a group of exercises. A *round* is completed by doing each exercise of a set in order, with appropriate rest times. Most exercises specify 30 seconds to one minute of rest after each round.

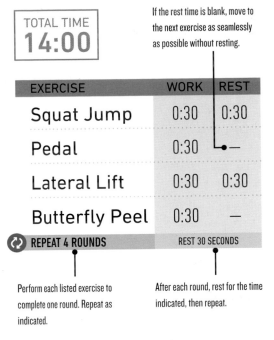

If the rest time is blank, move to the next exercise as seamlessly as possible without resting.

TOTAL TIME
14:00

EXERCISE	WORK	REST
Squat Jump	0:30	0:30
Pedal	0:30	—
Lateral Lift	0:30	0:30
Butterfly Peel	0:30	—

REPEAT 4 ROUNDS — REST 30 SECONDS

Perform each listed exercise to complete one round. Repeat as indicated.

After each round, rest for the time indicated, then repeat.

 TRAINER TIP

Be sure to have a watch or timer to measure these intervals, or use an app such as Interval Timer Pro.

LEARN THE EXERCISES

To keep HIIT interesting, you need a variety of effective and challenging exercises. This book includes step-by-step instructions for each of the 60 exercises used in the routines.

The exercises are grouped by primary focus (cardio, core, lower body, and upper body), but many challenge multiple muscle groups and provide cardiovascular benefits. Each exercise has a leveled progression guide, which provides alternate exercises for different ability levels. If you're feeling adventurous, try creating your own routines by combining several exercises.

TAKE A CHALLENGE

If you aren't sure where to start, check out the challenges at the end of each routines section. These programs give you a HIIT schedule to follow, from three days to four weeks. The routines are selected to increase in difficulty and intensity over time, leaving you stronger, fitter, and more toned at the end.

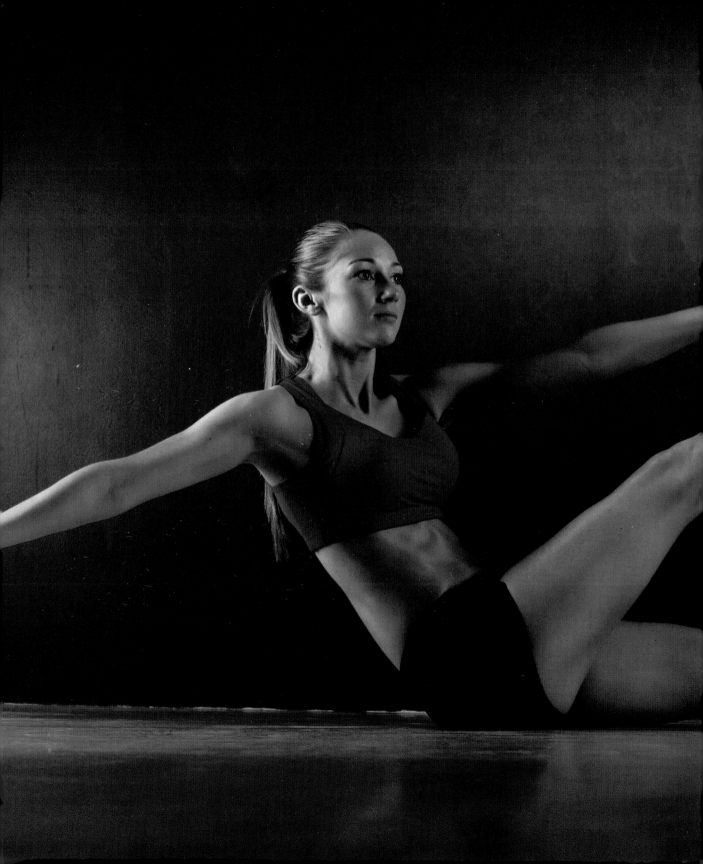

GETTING STARTED

HIIT is fast, flexible, and fun! In just minutes, you can get a workout that will fire up your metabolism, build strength, increase definition, and improve your health.

This part covers everything you need to know about HIIT: what it is, how it works, and how to maximize HIIT benefits through proper nutrition and recovery. Are you ready? Let's HIIT it!

WHAT IS HIIT?

High-intensity interval training, or HIIT, has exploded in recent years due to its promise of an efficient and effective way to meet fitness goals. Different trainers and instructors approach HIIT in different ways, but at its core, HIIT should always involve alternating short intervals of high-intensity, all-out exercise with short intervals of rest or active recovery.

What many people love about HIIT is that it's fast. You don't have to spend an hour at the gym every day. If you're willing to truly push yourself, you can get in an effective workout in just a few minutes.

ARE YOU WORKING HARD ENOUGH?

Because maximum effort is so critical to HIIT success, my clients often ask, "How do I know if I am working hard enough?" A good way to think about it is by measuring your workout intensity on a scale of 1 to 10, with 10 equal to running for your life. You should be working almost that hard during a HIIT workout, pushing yourself to a level 8 or 9. Remember that HIIT is hard. Your heart should be pounding, your breathing should be heavy, and you should be sweating.

HOW HIIT WORKS

Although short in duration, HIIT has a big impact. Training at your maximum capacity for intense intervals interspersed with rest or active recovery both accelerates fat loss and improves aerobic and anaerobic endurance.

HIGH INTENSITY

The "high intensity" part of HIIT is key. You won't see results if you're not pushing yourself as hard as you possibly can during the "work" intervals of your HIIT routine. Studies have shown that just seven minutes of HIIT can create changes in your muscles at a molecular level that are comparable to what you might see after an hour or more of traditional steady-state cardio, such as jogging or biking. However, those changes are not apparent if you don't work at maximum output.

CONSTANT CHANGE

The "interval" part of HIIT is also critical. This comes into play with both the brief rest periods between exercises as well as the order of exercises themselves. As you go through a HIIT routine, you alternate between periods of all-out exertion and active recovery or rest. The brief rest periods allow your heart rate to come down and prevent your body from adapting to a steady workload.

THE "AFTER BURN" EFFECT

Not only will you burn calories and fat during your HIIT workout, you will also burn calories and fat following your workout through the "after burn" effect, or EPOC (excess post-exercise oxygen consumption). EPOC is the measurable increased rate of oxygen intake following strenuous activity intended to erase the body's oxygen debt.

In order to erase the oxygen debt, fatty acids are released and used as fuel for recovery. You cannot take advantage of this after burn by doing low-intensity exercise. Only by working anaerobically at maximal heart rate will you see this added fat loss effect. EPOC has been shown to last over 48 hours.

EFFECTIVE EXERCISE COMBINATIONS

When it comes to HIIT, the types of exercises you do and the order in which you do them is important. An effective HIIT routine combines several different types of exercises in a way that will maximize the effects of each. The goal is to stimulate as many muscles as possible during each routine without overloading a particular muscle group. Frequent elevation changes (for example, transitioning from push-ups to squat jumps) help to drive up the heart rate, while multiplanar exercises (such as the cross-country seal) improve balance and athletic coordination.

HIIT BENEFITS

HIIT may seem too good to be true. The idea that you can work out for a shorter period of time and see greater health gains than you would with a traditional workout is counterintuitive. However, scientific studies back up the results.

EFFECTIVE WEIGHT LOSS

One reason HIIT is so popular is that it promises measurable and sustainable weight loss. If you're willing to work hard and monitor your nutrition, HIIT really is more effective than other forms of exercise for losing weight. One 1994 study at Laval University in Quebec, Canada, found that HIIT was nine times more effective for losing fat than steady-state cardio, such as jogging. This is because HIIT burns fat not only while you're working out, but also for up to 48 hours after exercising.

FAST, FLEXIBLE, AND FUN

Most HIIT workouts last 30 minutes or less and can be done anywhere, making HIIT the perfect choice for those who don't have the time or opportunity to squeeze in a full hour at the gym every day. With HIIT you have dozens of exercises to choose from that can be combined in countless ways. The ever-changing format of these HIIT routines will provide a unique and fun stimulus.

HIIT is also flexible; it can be done anywhere and requires no equipment. The exercises in this book rely on body weight resistance with an emphasis on achieving maximal heart rate.

LOSE FAT, NOT MUSCLE

If you've ever dieted, you know it's hard not to lose muscle mass along with fat. Studies show that HIIT workouts allow the preservation of muscle mass while losing weight through fat loss. This is because HIIT boosts testosterone and human growth hormone (HGH) levels, which are responsible for lean muscle gain and fat loss. HIIT stimulates the production of HGH by up to 450 percent during the 24 hours after you finish your workout. HGH is not only responsible for increasing your metabolism and stoking your fat-burning furnace; it also slows down the aging process.

IMPROVED HEART HEALTH

Pushing yourself into an anaerobic zone, where it feels like your heart is beating out of your chest, can actually improve your aerobic and anaerobic endurance. A 2012 study published in the *Journal of Strength and Conditioning Research* found that just six HIIT workouts performed over two or three weeks, each lasting only a few minutes, produced measurable improvements in key markers of cardiovascular health.

MITOCHONDRIAL GROWTH

The mitochondria are the power plants of your cells. These tiny cellular structures supply the cell's energy and are also involved with regulating cell growth. How does this relate to HIIT? In 2012, the *American Journal of Physiology* published an article stating that HIIT triggers mitochondrial biogenesis, the process by which new mitochondria are formed within a cell. Mitochondrial biogenesis begins to decline with age, so the ability of HIIT to trigger this process could be described as age-defying.

This is not the first time researchers have linked exercise to mitochondrial changes. A 2011 review in *Applied Physiology, Nutrition and Metabolism* points out that exercise induces changes in mitochondrial enzyme content and activity, which can increase your cellular energy production and in so doing decrease your risk of chronic disease. Mitochondrial changes may also benefit your liver, brain, and kidneys.

WHAT YOU NEED

One of the best things about HIIT is that you need little more than your body and a great attitude to get an incredible workout. However, there are a few pieces of equipment that will help to optimize your comfort and performance.

FOOTWEAR

During your workout, it's important to consider the placement of your feet on the floor. Improper positioning can lead to an unstable base of support and could cause injury.

To make you more aware of your foot position, I recommend a minimalist-style shoe when training. Two styles specifically designed for HIIT are the Nike Free 1.0 Cross Bionic and INOV-8's F-Lite range of shoes. If you're new to minimalist footwear, it's best to alternate between your old shoes and the minimalist shoes for about two weeks, allowing your body to adjust to the decrease in cushioning and support.

TOWEL

HIIT can get sweaty! Have a towel on hand to wipe the sweat from your brow and to keep your work surface dry.

FOAM ROLLER

Foam rollers are an inexpensive tool used to provide myofascial release in much the same way as static stretching and massage. Use of a foam roller can prevent injury and speed recovery post-workout.

YOGA MAT

You may wish to use a yoga mat for floor exercises. It will provide traction and may be more comfortable for exercises done on the back.

WATCH OR TIMER

A watch or timer is essential for keeping track of the work and rest intervals during HIIT routines. Use whatever is comfortable and easy to operate, whether it's a sport watch, a heart rate monitor, or a smartphone app that allows you to program intervals.

OPTIONAL EXTRAS

Some exercises can be made more challenging with the addition of a stability ball or gliding discs. Make sure you've mastered the movement before adding these options.

HIIT is about using as many muscle groups as possible in unison during fast explosive exercises. Adding weights or performing isolation exercises, such as bicep curls, can be prohibitive. However, for some core exercises, it's okay to challenge yourself by incorporating added weight. You can add resistance to exercises like Russian twists, V-ups, and sprinter sit-ups by using a dumbbell, kettlebell, or medicine ball.

In the studio I use a product called SandBells® from Hyperwear (hyperwear.com). These weights contain sand, which shifts with your movements, challenging your balance and making your workout more effective. Hyperwear also makes a product called Hyper-Vest® Pro. This weighted vest adds 10 pounds of evenly distributed weight to the torso, and is a safe and effective way to add resistance to every exercise in this book.

FITNESS ASSESSMENT

Before you get into HIIT, you need to assess your current fitness level. This simple fitness assessment will let you know where to start and give you a baseline for measuring your progress.

The fitness assessment consists of four basic exercises: X-jacks, push-ups, squats, and sprinter sit-ups. Before you begin, review the instructions for each exercise. Then complete these steps:

1. Do each exercise for 30 seconds.

2. Rest for 30 seconds after each exercise.

3. Record the number of reps you were able to do of each exercise during the 30-second interval (for example, 20 squats).

4. Add up the total number of reps completed for all exercises to get your total score.

EXERCISE	REPS COMPLETED
X-Jack	
Push-Up	
Squat	
Sprinter Sit-Up	
TOTAL:	

IF YOUR SCORE IS...	
0-80	Begin with the Level 1 routines.
81-104	Begin with the Level 2 routines.
105+	Begin with the Level 3 routines.

Use this assessment as a tool to track your progress and to know when you're ready to tackle the next level by reassessing every 14 days.

BODY FAT PERCENTAGE

HIIT is scientifically proven to burn body fat as well as generate lean muscle. Because muscle weighs more than fat, just tracking your weight may be a poor indication of your progress when undertaking HIIT. Calculating your body fat percentage can be a better way to measure results.

There are many different methods for measuring body fat, some more accurate than others. I advocate using a tape measure and the military method, which is the formula used by the U.S. Department of Defense for measuring body fat percentage.

 CAUTION

Although knowing your body fat percentage can help you determine realistic goals, keep in mind that it is just one of many ways to set goals and measure your fitness. Don't become obsessed with body fat percentage or any other measurement.

GET YOUR MEASUREMENTS

Use a tape measure to record the circumference of your neck, waist, and hips. Measure in inches or centimeters.

Neck. Measure your neck circumference at a point just below the larynx (Adam's apple) and perpendicular to the long axis of the neck. Round the measurement up to the nearest half inch (or half centimeter).

Waist. Measure your natural waist circumference, against the skin, at the narrowest point of the abdomen. This is usually about halfway between the navel and the lower end of the sternum (breast bone). Be sure the tape is level and parallel to the floor. Round the measurement down to the nearest half inch (or half centimeter).

Hip. Measure your hip circumference, passing the measuring tape over the fullest part of the glutes as viewed from the side. Make sure the tape is level and parallel to the floor. Round the hip measurement down to the nearest half inch (or half centimeter).

You will also need to know your height in inches or centimeters.

CALCULATE YOUR BODY FAT

To calculate your body fat percentage, plug your measurements into an online calculator: corepilatesandfitness.com/page18/index.html

You can also find your body fat percentage using the following formulas and a calculator with the LOG function.

For measurements in inches:

$$\text{Body fat percentage} = 163.205 \times \text{LOG}(\text{abdomen} + \text{hip} - \text{neck}) - 97.684 \times \text{LOG}(\text{height}) - 78.387$$

For measurements in centimeters:

$$\text{Body fat percentage} = 163.205 \times \text{LOG}(\text{abdomen} + \text{hip} - \text{neck}) - 97.684 \times \text{LOG}(\text{height}) - 104.912$$

Percent Body Fat Norms for Men and Women

	ESSENTIAL FAT	ATHLETIC	FIT	ACCEPTABLE	OBESE
Women	10–13%	14–20%	21–24%	25–31%	> 32%
Men	2–5%	6–13%	14–17%	18–24%	> 25%

From the American Council on Exercise.

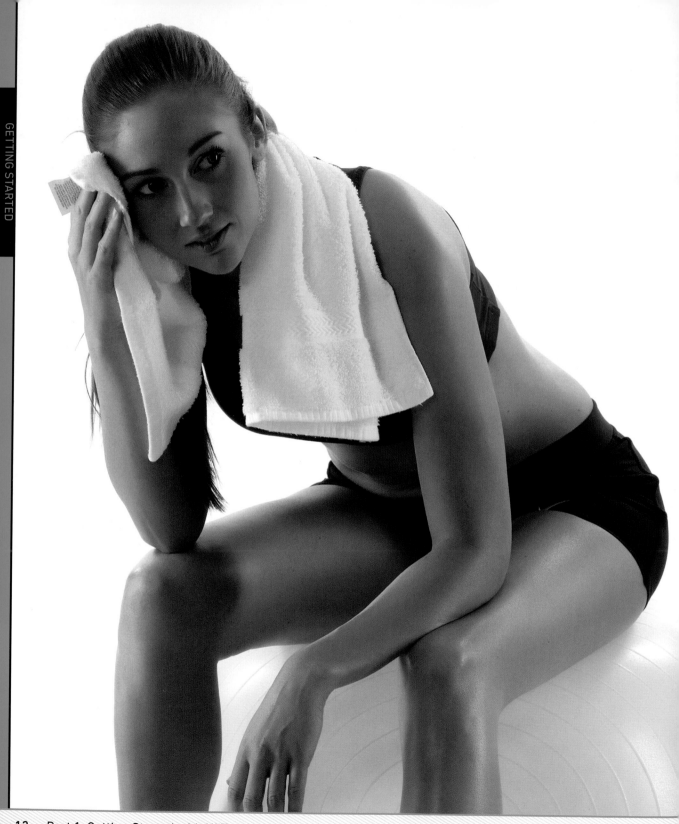

GOALS

Developing sound goals is critical to your HIIT performance. If you want to see long-term, sustainable success, then you need to be clear about what you want to accomplish. Successful goal setting requires SMART goals. Keep this acronym in mind when you consider what you want to achieve.

Once you've made your goals, help yourself stick to them by writing them down, making a plan to achieve them, and sharing them with friends and family. Be prepared for setbacks, and don't let minor slip ups cause you to lose focus.

SMART GOALS ARE...

Specific.
Simply and clearly define what you are going to do.

✓ "My goal is to perform 20 push-ups in 30 seconds."

✗ "My goal is to get better at push-ups."

Measurable.
You should be able to provide tangible evidence that you have met your goal.

✓ "My goal is to finish a 5K race in 21 minutes."

✗ "My goal is to run faster."

Achievable.
Make goals that are both challenging and realistic.

✓ "My goal is to lose 10 pounds in six weeks."

✗ "My goal is to lose 30 pounds in six weeks."

Results-driven.
Goals should be relevant and measure outcomes, not activities.

✓ "My goal is to burn 500 calories at the gym today."

✗ "My goal is to go to the gym."

Time-bound.
Goals should be linked to a time frame that creates a practical sense of urgency. Give yourself a deadline.

✓ "My goal is to lose 15 pounds in three months."

✗ "My goal is to lose 15 pounds."

DIET AND NUTRITION

Successful high-intensity interval training requires proper nutrition to ensure your body has enough fuel to power you through the HIIT workout.

BEFORE YOUR WORKOUT

As you go through a routine, your body uses stored glycogen along with carbohydrates ingested before the workout for fuel. A typical pre-HIIT meal should be light and provide a good balance of carbs and protein to fuel your workout. Don't eat anything too heavy or large; make this pre-workout snack approximately 200 to 300 calories.

AFTER YOUR WORKOUT

Post workout, it is important to replenish your body with protein and carbohydrates to aid in the repair and recovery process. Within 30 minutes of completing a HIIT workout, try to eat a meal that includes complex carbohydrates and a high protein content, such as $\frac{1}{3}$ cup cooked brown rice or quinoa, 1 cup cooked vegetables (2 cups raw), and 3 to 5 ounces lean meat. The carbohydrates will replenish the main source of fuel for your muscles, glyocen, and the antioxidants and protein in the meat will aid in the repair of muscle damage.

DURING THE DAY

You'll get the most out of your HIIT workouts if you eat simple, balanced meals in reasonable portions. I suggest eating lean meat, seafood, vegetables, fruits, whole grains, beans, low-fat dairy food, and healthy mono-saturated fats such as nuts, avocados, and olive oil. I also recommend avoiding sugar and processed foods. This is an eating plan that works for everyone, just adjust the serving sizes according to your needs.

HYDRATING

Proper hydration is vital to your athletic performance and health. To perform your best, you need to take in an adequate amount of fluid before, during, and after your workouts.

Thirty minutes before your workout, consume 5 to 10 ounces of a sports drink that is high in electrolytes such as sodium, potassium, magnesium, and chloride. Your hydration needs during your workout will depend on the duration and intensity of your activities. Always have water available and drink when you need to while working out.

FOR WEIGHT LOSS

If weight loss is your goal, you need to be aware of your caloric intake. HIIT provides a great fat-burning workout, but at the end of the day, weight loss comes down to a very simple equation: calories in versus calories out. The quality of those calories is also important. While diet choices are a personal decision, I advocate following a few simple guidelines if you're trying to lose weight.

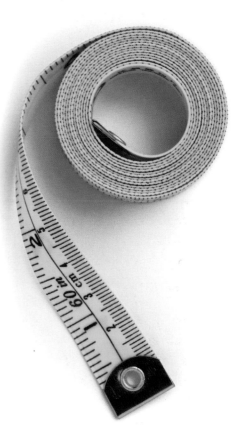

1 Eat three meals a day.

2 Eat two to three smaller snacks between meals, such as protein shakes, raw vegetables, or almonds. These snacks should be 100 to 200 calories.

3 Make sure your meals and snacks contain a good source and supply of lean protein. It's the building block of muscle.

4 Avoid foods made with white sugar and flour. Following this rule of thumb will help you stay away from the highly processed, simple carbohydrates that the body quickly turns to fat.

5 Cut out alcohol.

6 Limit your carbohydrates to unprocessed, complex carbs, such as sweet potatoes.

7 Eliminate soda, sweetened coffee beverages, and other high-calorie, sugary drinks.

8 Drink lots of water. It will help flush toxins from your body and keep you feeling satiated.

RECOVERY

HIIT requires you to push yourself to the limit during your workout, which means you need to allow time for rest and recovery. Recovery is critical for injury prevention and consistent training, and it enables you to give maximal effort each time you work out.

HYDRATION AND NUTRITION

Make sure you're getting the hydration and nutrition you need to fuel your HIIT workouts. Dehydration will reduce your performance and delay your recovery, so it's critical to replace your fluids and electrolytes.

What you eat is also important. Protein is the building block of new muscle and is required to rebuild muscle tissue. Carbohydrates replenish your glycogen stores and supply your muscles with energy. Be sure to get enough of each.

USING A FOAM ROLLER

A key component of recovery is self-myofascial release using a foam roller. The *fascia* is connective tissue that wraps around the muscles in the body. This tissue can become tense or constricted while working out, causing pain.

Using a foam roller to "roll out" the muscles can alleviate soreness and stiffness, promote circulation of oxygenated blood, and even break up scar tissue and restrictions in the fascia. A foam roller also allows you to apply targeted pressure to specific spots in the muscle that may be causing pain.

Look for a high-density foam roller that is about three inches (7.5 cm) in diameter. These can easily be found at sporting goods stores or online.

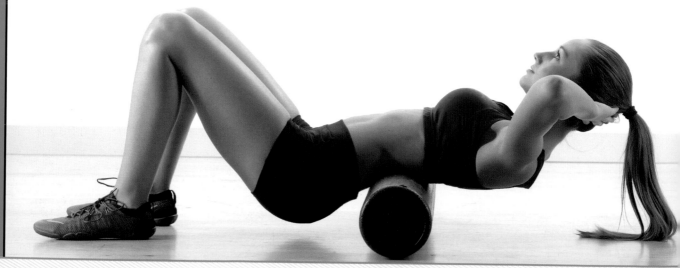

FOAM ROLLING TECHNIQUE

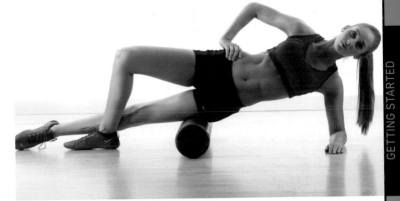

The foam roller can be used on many parts of the body, including the legs, back, and arms. The basic technique is the same, regardless of the area you're targeting. Use the roller as a warm-up, after working out, or whenever you feel pain.

1. Position your body on the roller. The weight of your body will apply pressure on your muscles. Roll back and forth slowly. When you find a tender spot in the area you are working, pause and wait for the discomfort to diminish. This could take up to one minute and may be uncomfortable.

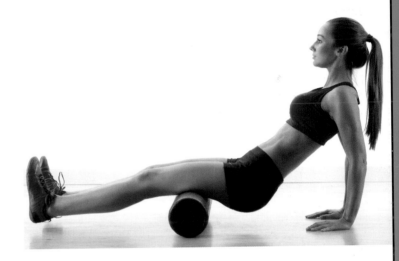

2. When the area is no longer sensitive, begin to roll up or down the muscle on the roller. Identify any other sensitive spots and repeat.

3. When tender areas can be rolled over without pain, continue rolling regularly to keep the area relaxed.

There is a lot of freedom for experimentation and "feel" when using the roller. See what works best for you and manipulate the roller to the correct position. You can create your own techniques to meet your needs.

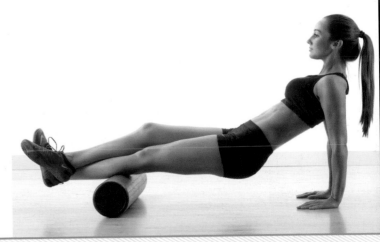

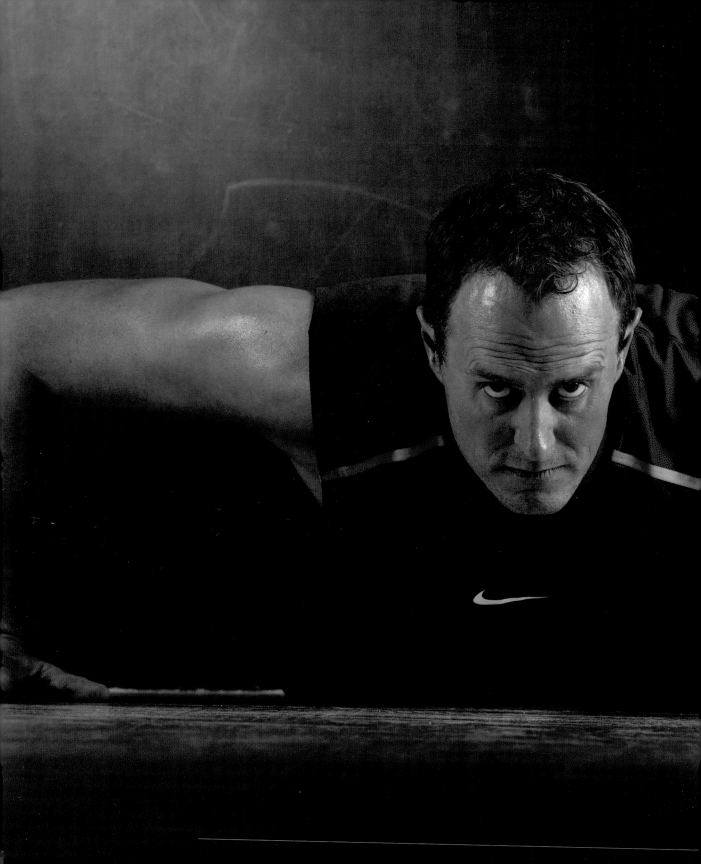

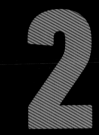

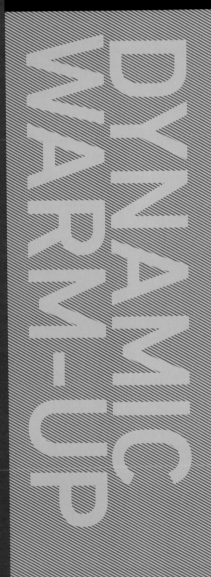

DYNAMIC WARM-UP

It's important to begin each HIIT workout with a dynamic warm-up. Unlike static stretching, dynamic stretching incorporates movement to activate the muscles you will use during your workout, improving your range of motion and challenging your balance and coordination. Dynamic stretching before a workout can help you lift more weight and increase overall athletic performance compared to no stretching or static stretching. If you are trying to become stronger, build more muscle, or simply perform better, a dynamic warm-up routine will help you meet your goal.

Complete each of the six warm-up exercises in this part in order, paying particular attention to form.

INNER THIGH MOBILITY

Warm up the hips and groin with this simple yet highly effective mobilization exercise.

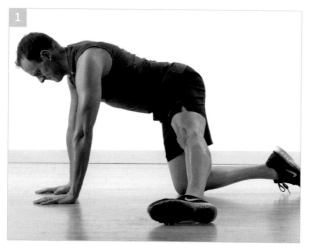

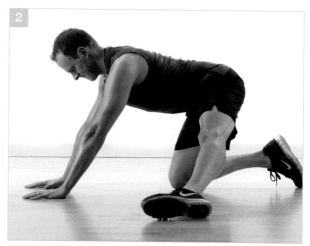

Begin on your hands and knees. Straighten your right leg out to the side until it is perpendicular to your torso.

Keep your back flat and push your hips back as far as possible.

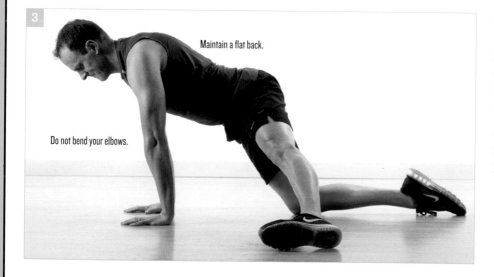

Maintain a flat back.

Do not bend your elbows.

Push your hips forward as far as you can, keeping your back flat and arms straight. Return to the starting position to complete one rep.

Complete 4 to 6 reps and then repeat with your left leg.

PEEL WITH REACH

The peel, or bridge position, is a great way to open your hips, activate your glutes, and engage your core, including the lower back. The addition of a reach aids in shoulder mobility.

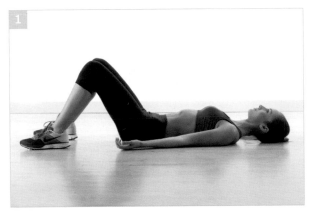

Lie on your back with knees bent at 90 degrees and feet flat on the floor. Spread your arms on the floor 45 degrees from your torso with palms facing up.

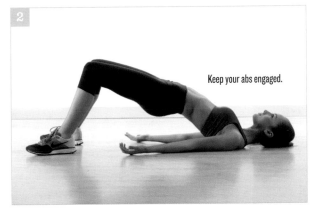

Keep your abs engaged.

Push through the heels and engage the glutes to lift the hips until your body forms a straight line from knees to shoulders.

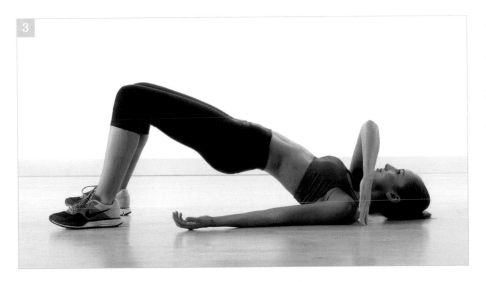

Holding the bridge position, lift your right arm and shoulder off the floor and reach across your torso to tap the floor behind your left shoulder.

Return to the starting position and perform 6 reps before repeating with your left arm.

HIP FLEXOR RELEASE TO WALKING LUNGE

Releasing your hip flexors will aid in hip mobility, ease back pain and tightness, and prepare you for exercises such as squats and pikes. Adding a walking lunge to activate the glutes, quads, and hamstrings makes this is a must-do warm-up before undertaking the explosive exercises of Levels 2 and 3.

TRAINER TIP

Pull knee as close to chest as possible, but remain tall through your torso.

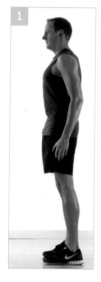

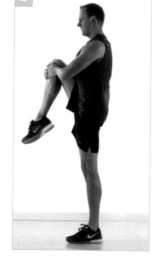

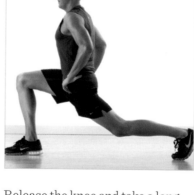

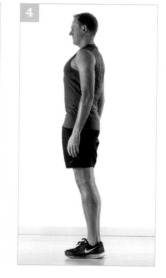

1 Stand with your feet hip width apart and arms at your sides.

2 Raise your right knee and grab just below the kneecap with both hands, pulling the knee toward your chest.

3 Release the knee and take a long stride forward with the right leg, lowering your body into a lunge with hands on hips or extended for stability.

4 Bring the back leg forward to meet your right and repeat with left leg.

Alternate for 5 per leg, 10 reps total.

CALF AND ANKLE MOBILITY

HIIT workouts often feature plyometric movements (jumping) and frequent changes of direction. It's important to keep your ankles, calves, and lower legs mobile to avoid injury and dysfunction.

TRAINER TIP

Slow down! Aim for maximum range of motion, not speed.

Begin in a standard push-up position. Lift your hips and place your left shin over your right calf muscle.

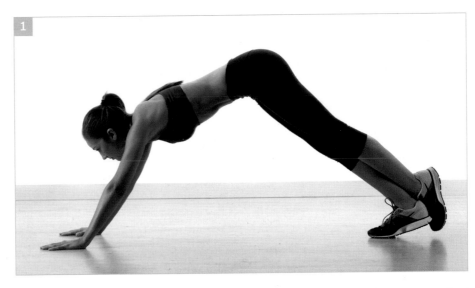

Slowly rock your hips back as if trying to make your heel touch the floor, and then forward onto the toes.

Perform 10 slow reps and then repeat on the left side.

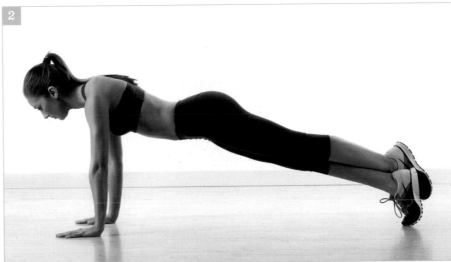

UPPER BACK ROTATION

Improve your posture by increasing the mobility in your thoracic spine with this simple exercise. It's especially beneficial for those who spend a lot of time at a desk or keyboard before starting HIIT.

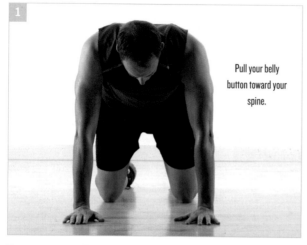

1

Pull your belly button toward your spine.

Begin on your hands and knees, with a flat back and straight arms.

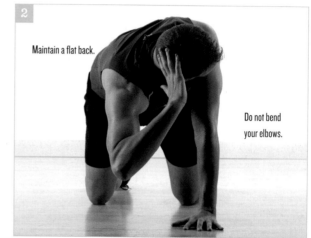

2

Maintain a flat back.

Do not bend your elbows.

Bring your right hand behind your head and rotate your right elbow inward toward the floor.

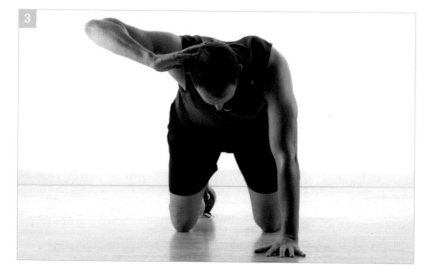

3

Reverse by rotating the right elbow outward to the ceiling, opening your chest and rotating your head and upper back as far as you can.

Rotate back inward and repeat for 8 reps before switching sides.

KNEELING PUSH-UP

Kneeling push-ups are a great way to warm up your chest, back, and shoulders and are also incredibly effective at activating the core and increasing shoulder stability.

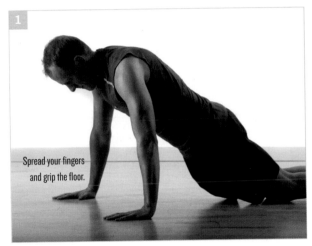

Spread your fingers and grip the floor.

Begin on all fours with your shoulders directly over your wrists. Tilt your pelvis and lower your hips until your body forms a straight line from knees to shoulders.

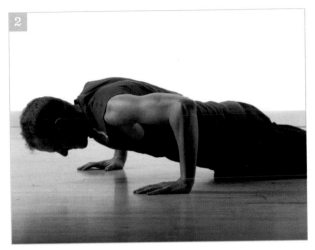

Bend your elbows, bringing your chest toward the floor. When your elbows are bent slightly beyond 90 degrees, hold for one to two seconds.

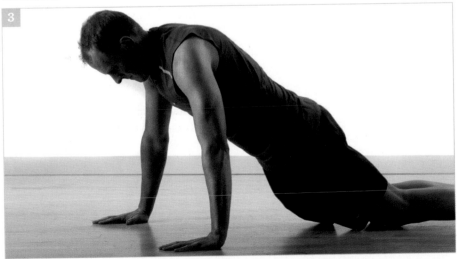

Push up through your palms, extending the arms to return to the starting position. Perform 10 reps, focusing on depth and range of motion.

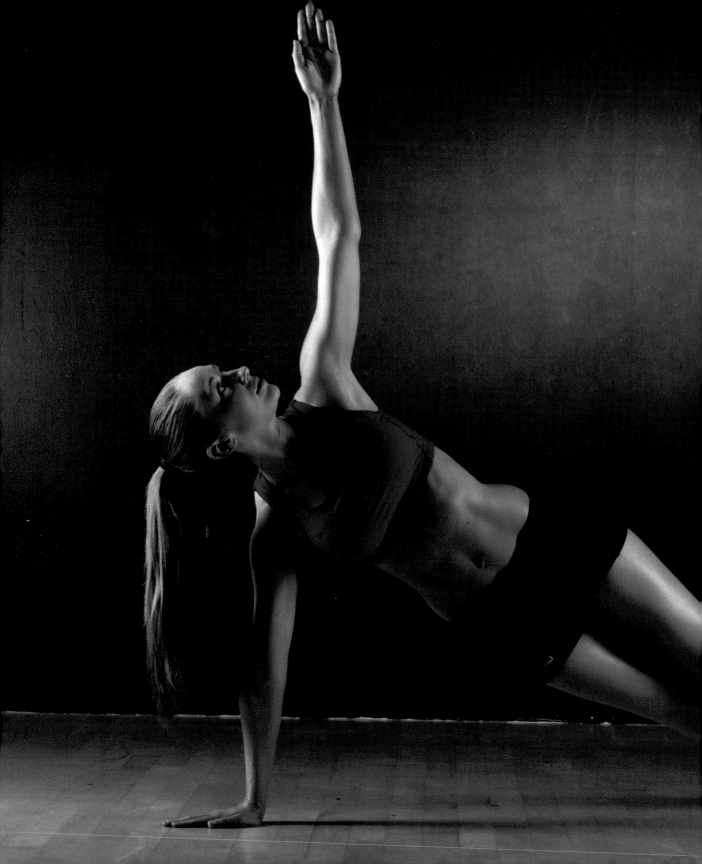

LEVEL 1 ROUTINES

Level 1 routines are designed to get you started with HIIT by introducing basic exercises and common routine formats in a way that is varied and challenging without being overwhelming. Level 1 gets things rolling with lower impact exercises, shorter routines, and longer rest periods. Remember the golden rule during each of these routines: form first and speed second.

No routine in Level 1 is longer than 20 minutes, and each has a work-to-rest ratio between 1:1 and 3:1. Try one on its own as a standalone introduction to HIIT, or choose one as a "finisher" at the end of a longer workout.

TOTAL TIME
5:00

FAST FIVES

Short, sharp, and incredibly effective, each of these routines is five minutes long and features cardio and compound exercise classics such as sprints and squats to charge your metabolism and burn calories.

 CHALLENGE

Try combining Routines A and B to create a 10-minute workout, or combine all four Fast Fives for a 20-minute workout.

ROUTINE A

Do each exercise for 20 seconds, followed by a 10-second rest. Rest 30 seconds after each round.

EXERCISE	WORK	REST
Sprint	0:20	0:10
Squat	0:20	0:10
Jumping Jack	0:20	0:10
Kneeling Push-Up	0:20	0:10
REPEAT 2 ROUNDS		REST 30 SECONDS

ROUTINE B

Do each exercise for 20 seconds, followed by a 10-second rest. Rest 30 seconds after each round.

EXERCISE	WORK	REST
High Knees	0:20	0:10
Reverse Lunge	0:20	0:10
Mountain Climber	0:20	0:10
Bicycle Crunch	0:20	0:10
REPEAT 2 ROUNDS		REST 30 SECONDS

TRAINER TIP

Fast Fives also make a great metabolic booster or "finisher" to other workouts. Try adding one to the end of a weight lifting session to super-charge your routine.

ROUTINE C

Do each exercise for 20 seconds, followed by a 10-second rest. Rest 30 seconds after each round.

EXERCISE	WORK	REST
Squat	0:20	0:10
Lunge	0:20	0:10
Lateral Lunge	0:20	0:10
Pelvic Peel	0:20	0:10
REPEAT 2 ROUNDS	REST 30 SECONDS	

ROUTINE D

Do each exercise for 20 seconds, followed by a 10-second rest. Rest 30 seconds after each round.

EXERCISE	WORK	REST
Pike	0:20	0:10
Bicycle Crunch	0:20	0:10
Circles	0:20	0:10
Plank	0:20	0:10
REPEAT 2 ROUNDS	REST 30 SECONDS	

THREE-PEAT

You'll discover that three really is the magic number in this total body challenge: three rounds, each with an increasing difficulty level and work-to-rest ratio. Each set blends high-output cardio with basic strength exercises.

Do each exercise in order, followed by the specified rest. Rest 30 seconds after each round.

EXERCISE	ROUND 1		ROUND 2		ROUND 3	
	WORK	REST	WORK	REST	WORK	REST
Sprint	0:15	0:15	0:20	0:10	0:30	—
Squat	0:15	0:15	0:20	0:10	0:30	—
High Knees	0:15	0:15	0:20	0:10	0:30	—
Mountain Climber	0:15	0:15	0:20	0:10	0:30	—
	REST 30 SECONDS		REST 30 SECONDS		REST 30 SECONDS	

CHALLENGE

Stack the rounds: Do Round 1 one time, Round 2 two times, and Round 3 three times. (Total Time 15:00)

Triple it: Do each round three times. (Total Time 22:30)

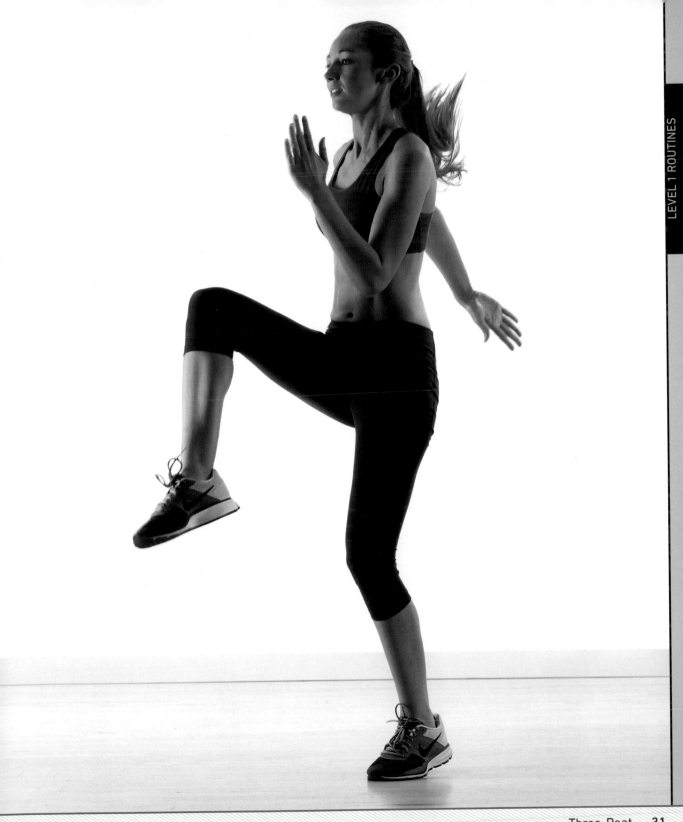

TOTAL TIME
10:00

HIIT OR QUIT

HIIT not only provides a physical challenge but improves mental toughness, requiring you to dig deep and push to maximal heart rate to achieve optimal results.

Do each exercise for 20 seconds. Rest one minute after each round.

EXERCISE	WORK	REST
Sprint	0:20	—
Jumping Jack	0:20	—
Squat Thrust	0:20	—
♻ REPEAT 5 ROUNDS		REST 1 MINUTE

TRAINER TIP

HIIT is all about maximal heart rate, so leave nothing in the tank. At the end of each set, you should be breathing hard and in need of rest. If you find the one-minute rest too long, cut it down to 30 seconds.

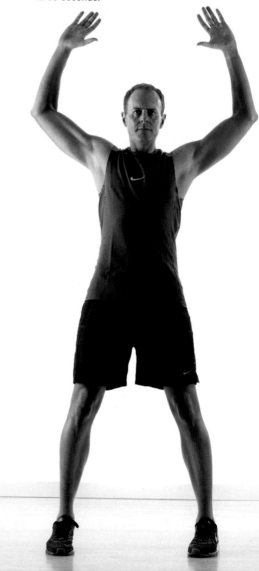

The change of elevation in this exercise forces your heart to work harder from battling the force of gravity. Remember: form first, speed second during this challenge. Good Luck!

Do as many squat thrusts as possible during each interval, followed by the specified rest. No rest between rounds.

EXERCISE	WORK	REST
Squat Thrust	0:30	0:15
Squat Thrust	0:30	0:30
Squat Thrust	0:30	0:15
⟳ REPEAT 2 ROUNDS	NO REST	

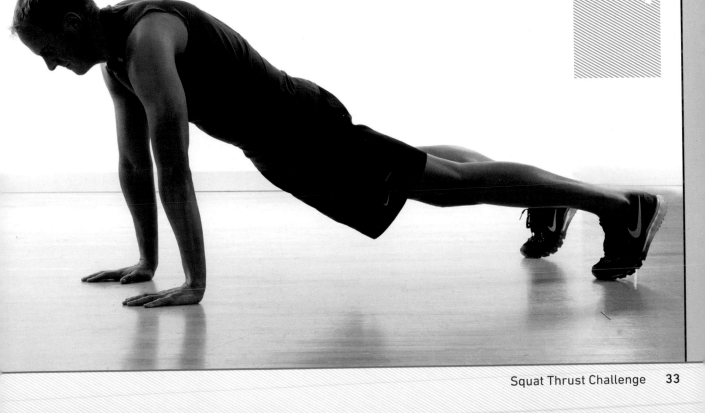

TOTAL TIME 10:00 — HIIT IT AGAIN

This simple, fun, and sweaty routine brings together three HIIT basics: sprints, squat thrusts, and mountain climbers. Push for maximum heart rate, and remember: you get out what you put in.

EXERCISE	WORK	REST
Squat Thrust	0:20	—
Mountain Climber	0:20	—
Sprint	0:20	—
REPEAT 5 ROUNDS		REST 1 MINUTE

Do each exercise in order. Rest one minute after each round.

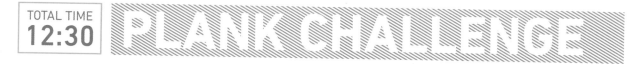

TOTAL TIME 12:30 — PLANK CHALLENGE

This deceptively simple exercise is the secret to rock-hard abs. The plank position engages the transverse abdominals, which aid in stabilization of the spine and pull in the tummy.

EXERCISE	WORK	REST
Plank	0:30	0:15
Plank	0:30	0:30
Plank	0:30	0:15
REPEAT 5 ROUNDS		NO REST

Hold a plank for as long as possible during each interval, followed by the specified rest. No rest between rounds.

TRAINER TIP

Be sure to maintain good form during your planks: elbows bent at 90 degrees, shoulders over elbows, head in line with the spine, and eyes over hands.

TOTAL TIME
15:00

CARDIO BURN

This routine combines explosive cardio elements, like sprinting, with large-muscle compound exercises, such as squats. The constant change of elevation between exercises makes you work harder than you might expect. You'll feel the burn after just one round.

Do each exercise for 20 seconds, followed by a 10-second rest. Rest one minute after each round.

EXERCISE	WORK	REST
Sprint	0:20	0:10
Squat	0:20	0:10
High Knees	0:20	0:10
Mountain Climber	0:20	0:10
Jumping Jack	0:20	0:10
Kneeling Push-Up	0:20	0:10
Shoulder Press Jack	0:20	0:10
Inchworm	0:20	0:10
↻ REPEAT 3 ROUNDS		REST 1 MINUTE

TOTAL TIME 21:00 HOT FOR HIIT

With each round of this challenging workout, the work-to-rest ratio increases. Varying the work-to-rest ratio and alternating exercises frequently keeps your body in a state of confusion, maximizing caloric burn and preventing it from adapting to a steady state.

Do each exercise in order, followed by the specified rest. Rest one minute after each round. Complete all three rounds.

EXERCISE	ROUND 1		ROUND 2		ROUND 3	
	WORK	REST	WORK	REST	WORK	REST
Jumping Jack	0:15	0:30	0:30	0:30	0:45	0:30
Kneeling Push-Up	0:15	0:30	0:30	0:30	0:45	0:30
Squat Thrust	0:15	0:30	0:30	0:30	0:45	0:30
T-Stand	0:15	0:30	0:30	0:30	0:45	0:30
Inchworm	0:15	0:30	0:30	0:30	0:45	0:30
Triceps Dip	0:15	0:30	0:30	0:30	0:45	0:30
	REST 1 MINUTE		REST 1 MINUTE		REST 1 MINUTE	

Work your biceps, triceps, shoulders, and back with these upper-body sculpting exercises. Build strength and definition while engaging the core and burning calories.

Do each exercise for 20 seconds, followed by a 10-second rest. Rest one minute after each round.

EXERCISE	WORK	REST
Side Press (right)	0:20	0:10
Inchworm	0:20	0:10
Side Press (left)	0:20	0:10
Kneeling Push-Up	0:20	0:10
↻ REPEAT 4 ROUNDS	REST 1 MINUTE	

TARGET: ARMS

TOTAL TIME
9:00

LEG HELL 1.0

This workout pushes your legs to the limit with a series of exercises targeting your calves, hamstrings, inner thighs, and glutes. Your legs will never be stronger, tighter, or more defined.

Do each exercise for 30 seconds. Rest one minute after each round.

EXERCISE	WORK	REST
Squat	0:30	—
Reverse Lunge	0:30	—
Lateral Lunge	0:30	—
T-Stand	0:30	—
REPEAT 3 ROUNDS		REST 1 MINUTE

TOTAL TIME
9:00

CORE KILLER

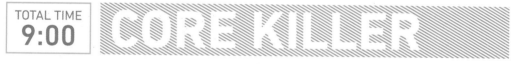

Each exercise in this series will challenge the muscles of the core (six-pack abs, obliques, transverse abs, back, and hips). A toned tummy may be your goal, but a stronger core will also improve athletic performance and balance.

Do each exercise for 30 seconds. Rest one minute after each round.

EXERCISE	WORK	REST
Bicycle Crunch	0:30	—
Pike	0:30	—
Circle (right)	0:30	—
Circle (left)	0:30	—
REPEAT 3 ROUNDS		REST 1 MINUTE

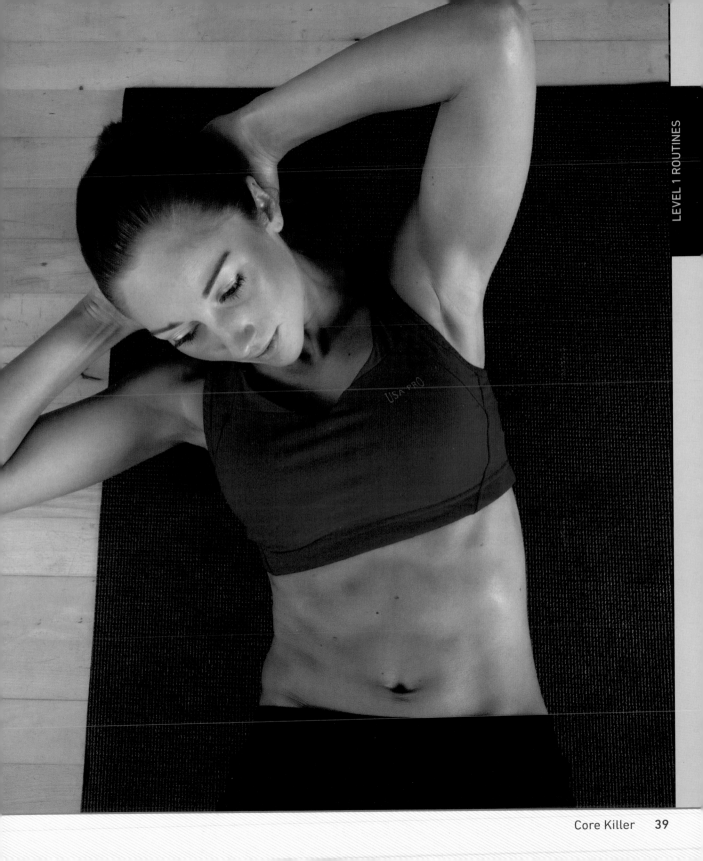

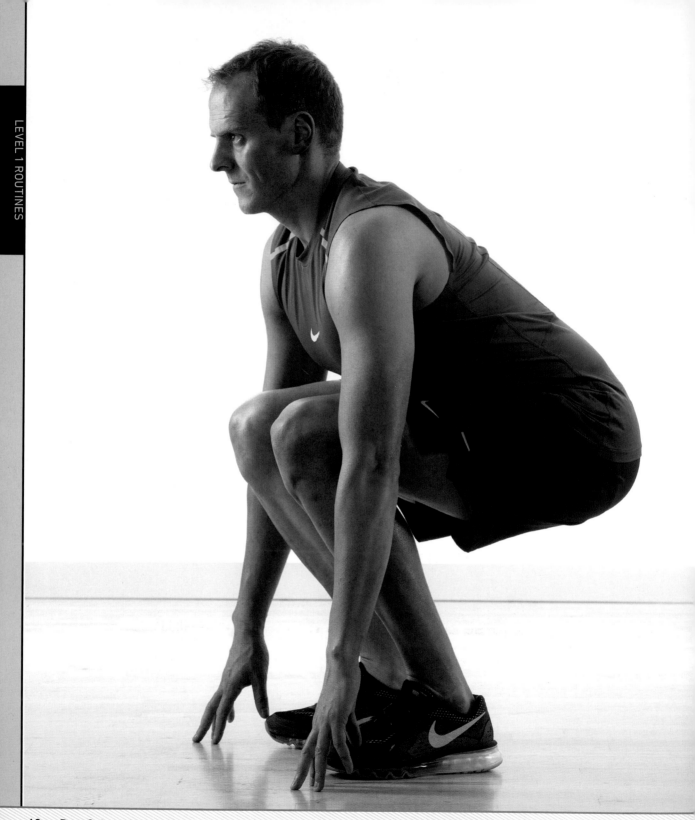

TOTAL TIME
20:00

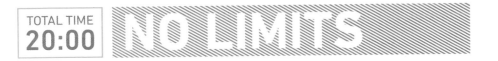
NO LIMITS

This metabolic-boosting routine is designed to push your limits. Give it all you have and work at maximal heart rate to extend the "after burn" effect of HIIT.

Do each exercise for 30 seconds, followed by a 30-second rest. Rest one minute after each round.

TRAINER TIP

If the 1:1 work-to-rest ratio provides too long a recovery, reduce the rest time to 15 seconds.

EXERCISE	WORK	REST
Sprint	0:30	0:30
Squat Thrust	0:30	0:30
High Knees	0:30	0:30
Plank	0:30	0:30
Pike	0:30	0:30
Bicycle Crunch	0:30	0:30
Squat	0:30	0:30
Reverse Lunge	0:30	0:30
Lateral Lunge	0:30	0:30
⟳ REPEAT 2 ROUNDS	REST 1 MINUTE	

TOTAL TIME
15:00

CUT TO THE CORE

The core muscles work as stabilizers for the entire body and help the body function more effectively. Strengthening these muscles will provide definition and improve athleticism and coordination.

Do each exercise for 20 seconds, followed by a 10-second rest. Rest one minute after each round.

EXERCISE	WORK	REST
Pike	0:20	0:10
Plank	0:20	0:10
Bicycle Crunch	0:20	0:10
Side Plank (right)	0:20	0:10
Circles (right)	0:20	0:10
Side Plank (left)	0:20	0:10
Circles (left)	0:20	0:10
Plank	0:20	0:10
REPEAT 3 ROUNDS		REST 1 MINUTE

FAT BURNER

TOTAL TIME 18:00

Short bursts of intense, heart-rate–boosting activity are coupled with classic strength exercises in this dynamic yet challenging routine. Burn calories, gain strength, and increase athletic performance in under 20 minutes!

Do each exercise for 20 seconds, followed by a 10-second rest. Rest 30 seconds after each round.

EXERCISE	WORK	REST
High Knees	0:20	0:10
Mountain Climber	0:20	0:10
Squat	0:20	0:10
Peel	0:20	0:10
Sprint	0:20	0:10
Kneeling Push-Up	0:20	0:10
Jumping Jack	0:20	0:10
Triceps Dip	0:20	0:10
REPEAT 4 ROUNDS	REST 30 SECONDS	

TRAINER TIP

When you only spend 18 minutes on a workout, you need to make every minute count. Keep the transitions between exercises as fast as possible to maximize your calorie-burning time.

TOTAL TIME	
16:30	# ENDURO

This routine challenges your endurance with longer cardio segments and greater muscular demands. Endurance-oriented routines are especially beneficial if you play sports that require sustained activity for a long period of time.

Do each exercise for 30 seconds. Rest one minute after each round.

EXERCISE	WORK	REST
Jumping Jack	0:30	—
Reverse Lunge	0:30	—
Inchworm	0:30	—
High Knees	0:30	—
Mountain Climber	0:30	—
Squat Thrust	0:30	—
Lateral Lunge	0:30	—
Kneeling Push-Up	0:30	—
Plank	0:30	—
⟳ **REPEAT 3 ROUNDS**	**REST 1 MINUTE**	

TRAINER TIP

It's okay to feel winded when performing HIIT. If you're working at your maximal heart rate, it will be uncomfortable and will take mental toughness to push through.

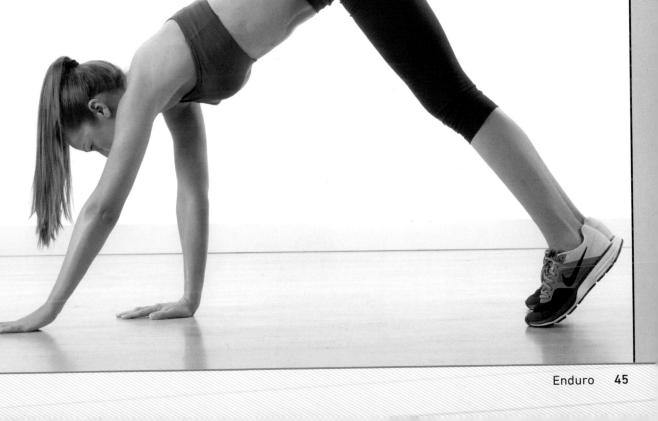

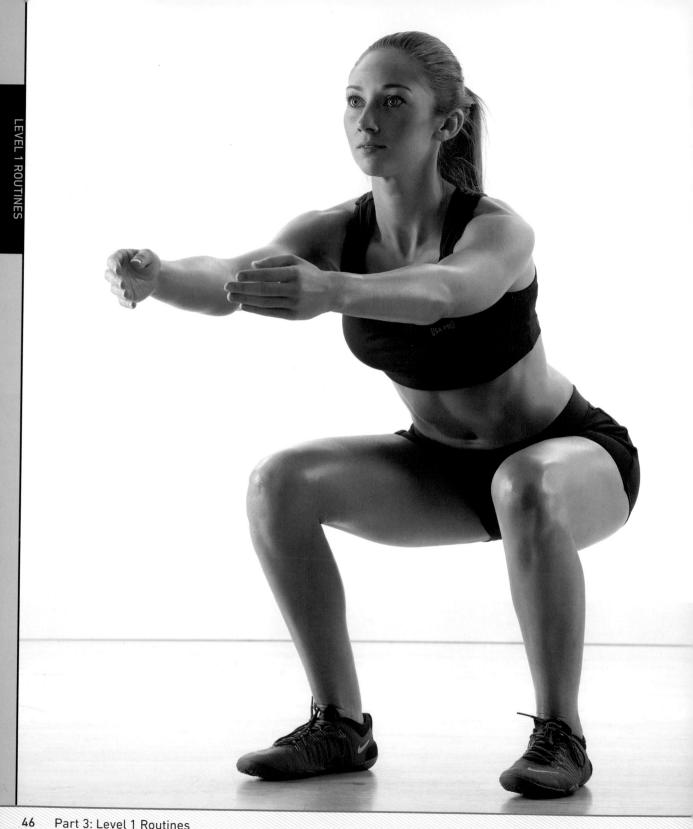

TOTAL TIME 10:00 — EVERY SECOND COUNTS

This short but incredibly effective routine will push you to your limits, elevate your heart rate, and burn calories.

Do each exercise for 20 seconds. Rest one minute after each round.

EXERCISE	WORK	REST
Jumping Jack	0:20	—
High Knees	0:20	—
Squat Thrust	0:20	—
⟳ REPEAT 5 ROUNDS		REST 1 MINUTE

TOTAL TIME 10:00 — TRIFECTA

The three simple exercises in this routine will activate the chest, back, quads, and glutes. These large muscle groups burn the most calories both when working and during recovery, making this a go-to routine if you are short on time but need big results.

Do each exercise for 20 seconds. Rest one minute after each round.

EXERCISE	WORK	REST
Sprint	0:20	—
Squat	0:20	—
Kneeling Push-Up	0:20	—
⟳ REPEAT 5 ROUNDS		REST 1 MINUTE

TOTAL TIME 9:30

SORE OR SORRY?

You can either wake up sore but satisfied, or you can wake up sorry that you didn't work out. The combination of cardio and strength exercises in this routine will deliver soreness—and satisfaction.

Do each exercise in order, followed by the specified rest. Rest one minute after each round. Complete both rounds.

EXERCISE	ROUND 1		ROUND 2	
	WORK	REST	WORK	REST
Sprint	0:15	0:15	0:30	0:15
Reverse Lunge	0:15	0:15	0:30	0:15
High Knees	0:15	0:15	0:30	0:15
T-Stand	0:15	0:15	0:30	0:15
Inchworm	0:15	0:15	0:30	0:15
Shoulder Press Jack	0:15	0:15	0:30	0:15
	REST 1 MINUTE		REST 1 MINUTE	

TOTAL TIME 12:00

CORE CHAOS

The plank position forces you to engage your deepest core muscles, strengthening the muscle groups that stabilize the spine (including your lower back and glutes) and improving your posture.

Do each round three times. Rest one minute after each round.

EXERCISE	ROUND 1		ROUND 2	
	WORK	REST	WORK	REST
Plank	0:20	—	0:10	—
Side Plank (right)	0:10	—	0:20	—
Plank	0:20	—	0:10	—
Side Plank (left)	0:10	—	0:20	—
⟳ REPEAT 3 ROUNDS	REST 1 MINUTE		REST 1 MINUTE	

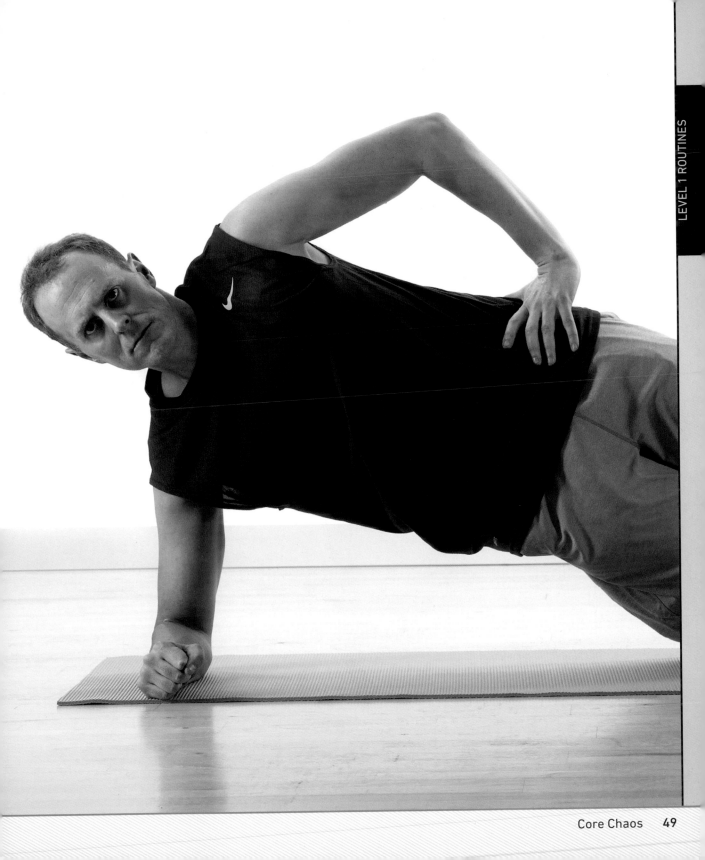

TOTAL BODY BLAST

This routine features a challenging series of compound, multi-muscle exercises. Each round has a different work-to-rest ratio to keep your body on its toes and guarantee results.

Do each exercise in order, followed by the specified rest. Rest one minute after each round.

EXERCISE	ROUND 1		ROUND 2		ROUND 3	
	WORK	REST	WORK	REST	WORK	REST
Jumping Jack	0:15	0:15	0:20	0:10	0:30	0:30
Squat	0:15	0:15	0:20	0:10	0:30	0:30
Kneeling Push-Up	0:15	0:15	0:20	0:10	0:30	0:30
Mountain Climber	0:15	0:15	0:20	0:10	0:30	0:30
Lateral Lunge	0:15	0:15	0:20	0:10	0:30	0:30
Triceps Dip	0:15	0:15	0:20	0:10	0:30	0:30
Squat Thrust	0:15	0:15	0:20	0:10	0:30	0:30
T-Stand	0:15	0:15	0:20	0:10	0:30	0:30
Plank	0:15	0:15	0:20	0:10	0:30	0:30
	REST 1 MINUTE		REST 1 MINUTE		REST 1 MINUTE	

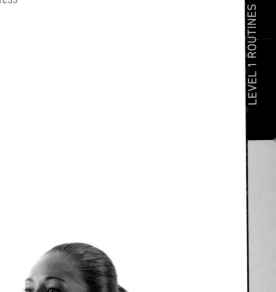

TRAINER TIP

During plank-oriented exercises, spread your fingers and
"claw" the floor to distribute weight and reduce stress
on wrists.

TOTAL TIME
16:00

JACKED

EXERCISE	WORK	REST
Jumping Jack	0:30	—
Shoulder Press Jack	0:30	—
⟳ **REPEAT 8 ROUNDS**		REST 1 MINUTE

Get jacked for this cardio routine featuring two different variations on the classic jumping jack. This workout will push your heart rate, burn fat, and improve athletic performance, agility, and foot speed.

Do each exercise for 30 seconds. Rest one minute after each round.

TOTAL TIME
13:30

STACKED

The change of elevation and fast-paced exercises in this routine will push your limits.

Do each exercise for 30 seconds, followed by the specified rest time. Rest 30 seconds after each round.

EXERCISE	WORK	REST
Sprint	0:30	0:30
Sprint	0:30	—
Squat Thrust	0:30	0:30
Sprint	0:30	—
Squat Thrust	0:30	—
Kneeling Push-Up	0:30	—
⟳ **REPEAT 3 ROUNDS**		REST 30 SECONDS

TONED ARMS

TOTAL TIME
15:00

This fast and effective routine isolates the muscles of the back, chest, shoulders, and triceps to sculpt, strengthen, and tone the upper body.

Do each exercise for 30 seconds. Rest one minute after each round.

EXERCISE	WORK	REST
Kneeling Push-Up	0:30	—
Side Press (right)	0:30	—
Triceps Dip	0:30	—
Side Press (left)	0:30	—
REPEAT 5 ROUNDS		REST 1 MINUTE

STRONG LEGS

TOTAL TIME
17:30

Stairs will be your enemy for a day or two after this strenuous routine, but the results will be worth it. These lower-body exercises will increase definition and build strength in your quads, lengthen your hamstrings, and firm and round your glutes.

Do each exercise for 20 seconds, followed by a 10-second rest. Rest 30 seconds after each round.

EXERCISE	WORK	REST
Squat	0:20	0:10
T-Stand (right)	0:20	0:10
Reverse Lunge	0:20	0:10
T-Stand (left)	0:20	0:10
Lateral Lunge	0:20	0:10
Pelvic Peel	0:20	0:10
REPEAT 5 ROUNDS		REST 30 SECONDS

TOTAL TIME 22:30 TRIPLE PLAY

This metabolic-boosting routine is designed to push your limits. Give it all you have and work at maximal heart rate to extend the "after burn" effect of HIIT.

Do each exercise for 20 seconds, followed by a 10-second rest. Do three rounds of each set before moving to the next. Rest 30 seconds after each round.

SET 1

EXERCISE	WORK	REST
High Knees	0:20	0:10
Squat Thrust	0:20	0:10
Mountain Climber	0:20	0:10
Sprint	0:20	0:10
REPEAT 3 ROUNDS		REST 30 SECONDS

SET 2

EXERCISE	WORK	REST
Squat	0:20	0:10
Reverse Lunge	0:20	0:10
Lateral Lunge	0:20	0:10
Pelvic Peel	0:20	0:10
REPEAT 3 ROUNDS		REST 30 SECONDS

SET 3

EXERCISE	WORK	REST
Kneeling Push-Up	0:20	0:10
Plank	0:20	0:10
Triceps Dip	0:20	0:10
Bicycle	0:20	0:10
REPEAT 3 ROUNDS		REST 30 SECONDS

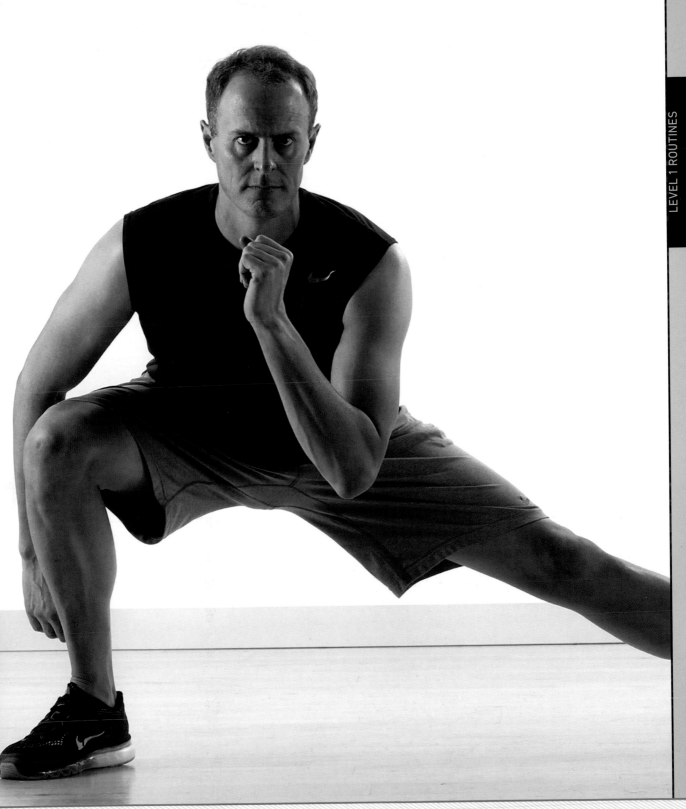

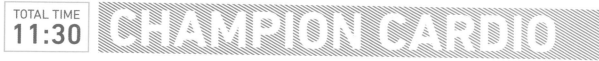

TOTAL TIME 11:30

CHAMPION CARDIO

Push to your limits with this high output, total-body routine geared for peak performance.

Do each exercise for 30 seconds, followed by a 10-second rest. Rest 30 seconds after each round.

EXERCISE	WORK	REST
High Knees	0:30	0:10
Squat Thrust	0:30	0:10
Mountain Climber	0:30	0:10
Sprint	0:30	0:10
Jumping Jack	0:30	0:10
REPEAT 3 ROUNDS		REST 30 SECONDS

TOTAL TIME 16:00

TARGET: ABS

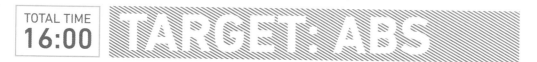

Sleek, sexy, defined abs require nutritional discipline and dedication to your training. The exercises in this routine lift, twist, and turn to activate muscle fibers and get results faster.

Do each exercise for 20 seconds, followed by a 10-second rest. Rest 30 seconds after each round.

EXERCISE	WORK	REST
Bicycle Crunch	0:20	0:10
Pike	0:20	0:10
Circles	0:20	0:10
REPEAT 8 ROUNDS		REST 30 SECONDS

TRAINER TIP

Change the direction of your circles with each round.

NO GRIND, NO GLORY

TOTAL TIME 12:00

Complete eight rounds of intense exercises that target your shoulders, back, core, and legs. You get what you earn with this routine.

Do each exercise for 20 seconds. Rest 30 seconds after each round.

EXERCISE	WORK	REST
Squat Thrust	0:20	—
Inchworm	0:20	—
Mountain Climber	0:20	—
↻ REPEAT 8 ROUNDS		REST 30 SECONDS

PUSH-UP INTERVALS

TOTAL TIME 7:00

The push-up builds upper body and core strength using the muscles of the chest, back, shoulders, triceps, abs, and even the legs. Keep an eye on your form.

Complete as many kneeling push-ups in each interval as possible, followed by the specified period of rest.

EXERCISE	WORK	REST
Kneeling Push-Up	0:10	0:10
Kneeling Push-Up	0:20	0:20
Kneeling Push-Up	0:20	0:10
Kneeling Push-Up	0:30	0:30
Kneeling Push-Up	0:20	0:20
Kneeling Push-Up	0:30	1:00
Kneeling Push-Up	0:20	0:20
Kneeling Push-Up	0:20	0:20
Kneeling Push-Up	0:10	0:10
Kneeling Push-Up	0:20	0:20

TRAINER TIP

To vary the muscle groups targeted during the kneeling push-ups, alternate your hand positions to include standard push-ups, military push-ups, and diamond push-ups. Each will activate a different area of the chest, back, and arms.

LEVEL 1 3-DAY CHALLENGE

If you're having trouble getting started with HIIT, challenge yourself to three days of workouts that include some popular HIIT basics. Each head-to-toe workout combines high-output cardio and compound strength exercises to give you a firm foundation for HIIT.

DAY	ROUTINE
1	Three-Peat
2	HIIT It Again
3	Triple Play

TRAINER TIPS

- To decrease the risk of injury and prepare yourself to perform at 100 percent, remember to warm up each day before beginning your HIIT routine.

- Focus on form before speed. Make sure you know how to do each exercise properly before beginning your routine.

- Stay hydrated and don't let your diet undo all your hard work! To get the results you want, you'll need to eat right.

If you'd like to lose a few pounds or shake up your regular workout routine, a week of HIIT can help. The 7-Day Challenge includes a variety of HIIT routine formats and features exercises designed to burn fat, lose weight, increase strength, and improve athletic performance.

DAY	ROUTINE
1	Three-Peat
2	Toned Arms
3	Cardio Burn
4	Cut to the Core
5	Enduro
6	Strong Legs
7	Triple Play

 TRAINER TIPS

- To perform your best and prevent injury, begin each routine with a dynamic warm up.

- The 7-Day Challenge introduces more athletic exercises, so form is more important than ever. Be sure you know how to do each exercise correctly before beginning your routine.

- Expect to be sore. If your workouts are as intense as they should be, you will be sore the next day. Remember that sore muscles are not the same as pain due to injury.

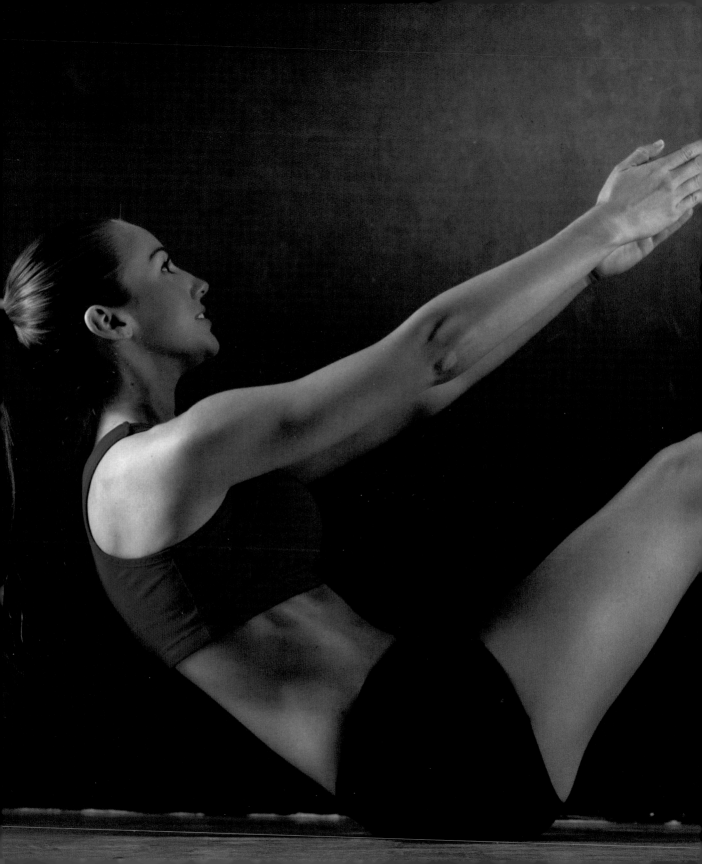

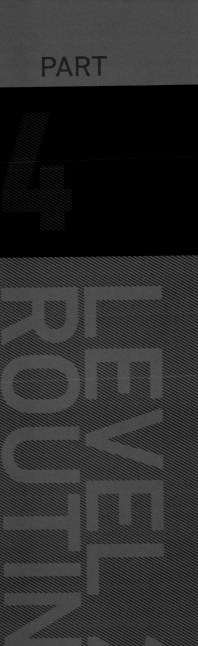

The Level 2 routines are more challenging than those for Level 1 and include plyometrics (jump training), frequent elevation changes, and an increased level of difficulty.

Level 2 routines range from 5 minutes to 40 minutes in length, with work-to-rest ratios between 2:1 and 4:1. Consider incorporating the shorter routines into a longer workout as a metabolic-boosting "finisher."

TOTAL TIME
15:00

NO EXCUSES

This high-energy routine features the X-jack and the cross-country seal, two plyometric exercises that that will challenge your cardiovascular output, strength, and coordination.

Do each exercise for 30 seconds. Rest 30 seconds after each round.

EXERCISE	WORK	REST
X-Jack	0:30	—
Cross-Country Seal	0:30	—
X-Jack	0:30	—
Cross-Country Seal	0:30	—
♻ REPEAT 6 ROUNDS	REST 30 SECONDS	

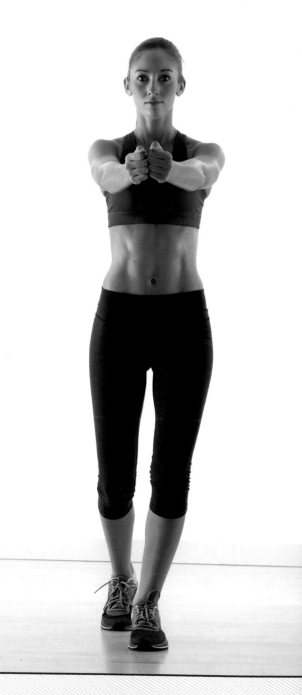

LEG HELL 2.0

TOTAL TIME
10:00

This workout pushes your legs to the limit with a series of exercises targeting your calves, hamstrings, inner thighs, and glutes. Your legs will never be stronger, tighter, or more defined.

Do each exercise for 30 seconds. Rest 30 seconds after each round.

EXERCISE	WORK	REST
Squat Jump	0:30	—
Pedal	0:30	—
Lateral Lift	0:30	—
Pigeon or Butterfly Peel	0:30	—
↻ REPEAT 4 ROUNDS		**REST 30 SECONDS**

TRAINER TIP

Alternate between pigeon and butterfly pelvic peels each round, completing a total of two rounds of each.

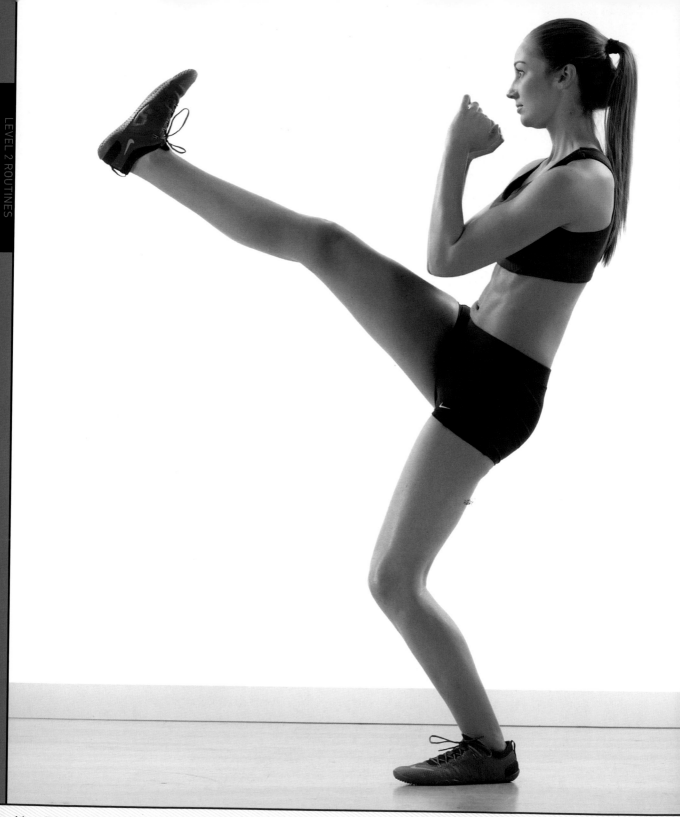

TOTAL TIME
30:00

FIRM AND BURN

This half-hour routine delivers a head-to-toe workout with an emphasis on calorie burning and compound (multi-muscle) exercises.

Do each set three times before moving to the next. Rest 30 seconds after each round.

SET 1

EXERCISE	WORK	REST
Cross-Country Seal	0:30	—
Push-Up	0:30	—
Pedal	0:30	—
Burpee	0:30	—

⟳ REPEAT 3 ROUNDS — REST 30 SECONDS

SET 2

EXERCISE	WORK	REST
Squat Jump	0:30	—
X-Jack	0:30	—
Diagonal Mountain Climber	0:30	—
Squat Hold	0:30	—

⟳ REPEAT 3 ROUNDS — REST 30 SECONDS

SET 3

EXERCISE	WORK	REST
V-Up	0:30	—
In-and-Out Abs	0:30	—
Spiderman	0:30	—
Tuck Jump	0:30	—

⟳ REPEAT 3 ROUNDS — REST 30 SECONDS

SET 4

EXERCISE	WORK	REST
T-Stand Kick (right)	0:30	—
Grasshopper	0:30	—
T-Stand Kick (left)	0:30	—
Shoulder Press	0:30	—

⟳ REPEAT 3 ROUNDS — REST 30 SECONDS

TOTAL TIME 10:00 HI-LOW

Plyometrics (jump training) is all about explosive power, balance, and agility. Changing the elevation of the body from high to low and back again ignites the body's fat-burning furnace and improves athletic performance in the process.

Do each exercise for 30 seconds. Rest 30 seconds after each round.

EXERCISE	WORK	REST
Burpee	0:30	—
X-Jack	0:30	—
Diagonal Mountain Climber	0:30	—
Squat Jump	0:30	—
⟳ REPEAT 4 ROUNDS		REST 30 SECONDS

TOTAL TIME 12:00 DOUBLE CROSS

These two exercises target the obliques, transverse abs, and six-pack abs, forcing you to stabilize your spine and support your body weight through your core as you rotate.

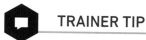

TRAINER TIP

Control your speed. Don't allow momentum to carry your movements. Move with purpose and poise.

Do each exercise for 30 seconds. Rest 30 seconds after each round.

EXERCISE	WORK	REST
Double-Cross Reach	0:30	—
Diagonal Mountain Climber	0:30	—
⟳ REPEAT 8 ROUNDS		REST 30 SECONDS

TOTAL TIME 10:00

JUMP FOR IT

Tuck jumps are one of the most challenging HIIT exercises, but they offer incredible benefits. The rapid plyometric movement sends your heart rate soaring, scorches calories, and can even improve bone density.

Do each exercise for 20 seconds, followed by a 10-second rest. Rest 30 seconds after each round.

EXERCISE	WORK	REST
Tuck Jump	0:20	0:10
Push-Ups	0:30	—
Tuck Jump	0:20	0:10
In-and-Out Abs	0:30	—
REPEAT 4 ROUNDS	REST 30 SECONDS	

TRAINER TIP

Keep your core engaged when doing tuck jumps, and land softly, bending at the ankles, knees, and hips to absorb your impact.

TOTAL TIME 9:00

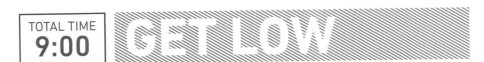

GET LOW

People often worry that deep squats may cause harm to their knees. In fact, deep squats are incredibly beneficial if done with proper form. Try to get as low as you can during this routine, but keep form in mind.

Do each exercise for 20 seconds. Rest 30 seconds after each round.

EXERCISE	WORK	REST
Squat	0:20	—
Reverse Lunge	0:20	—
Squat Jump	0:20	—
REPEAT 6 ROUNDS	REST 30 SECONDS	

TRAINER TIP

Dorsiflexion is the bending of the toes toward the shin. At the bottom of the squat, you should have roughly 15 degrees of dorsiflexion in your ankles. A low-profile minimalist shoe is helpful for achieving this bend.

TOTAL TIME 30:00 FIT FRENZY

This frenzied 30-minute routine delivers a head-to-toe workout with an emphasis on calorie-scorching plyometric exercises.

Do each exercise 30 seconds. Do three rounds of each set before moving to the next. Rest 30 seconds after each round.

SET 1

EXERCISE	WORK	REST
Burpee	0:30	—
Diagonal Mountain Climber	0:30	—
Pedal	0:30	—
Grasshopper	0:30	—
REPEAT 3 ROUNDS		REST 30 SECONDS

SET 2

EXERCISE	WORK	REST
V-Up	0:30	—
Double-Cross Reach	0:30	—
Russian Twist	0:30	—
Plank	0:30	—
REPEAT 3 ROUNDS		REST 30 SECONDS

SET 3

EXERCISE	WORK	REST
X-Jack	0:30	—
T-Stand Kick (right)	0:30	—
Tuck Jump	0:30	—
T-Stand Kick (left)	0:30	—
REPEAT 3 ROUNDS		REST 30 SECONDS

SET 4

EXERCISE	WORK	REST
Cross-Country Seal	0:30	—
Squat Jump	0:30	—
Military Push-Up	0:30	—
In-and-Out Abs	0:30	—
REPEAT 3 ROUNDS		REST 30 SECONDS

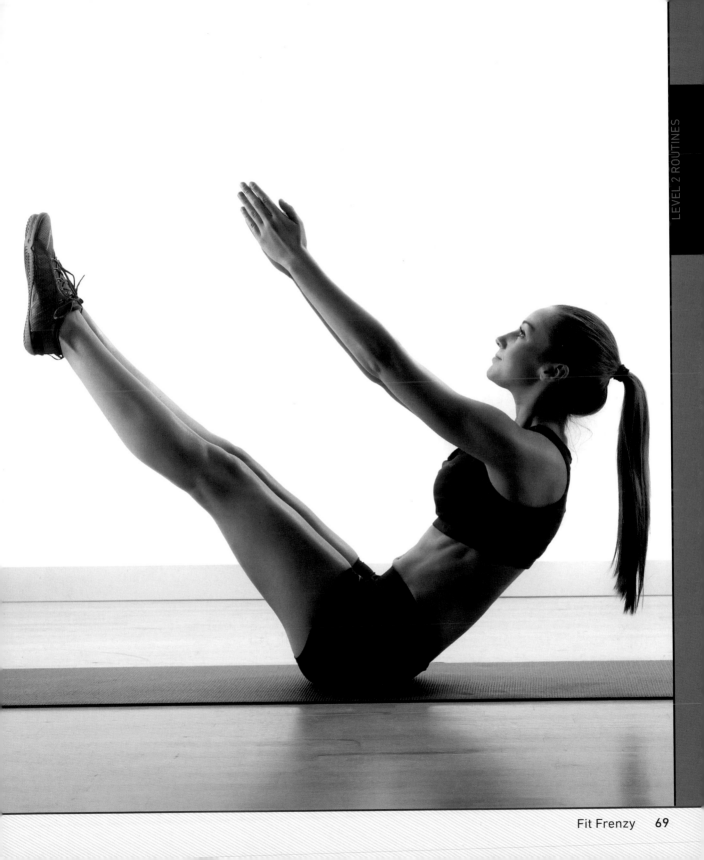

TOTAL TIME 12:00 HARD CORE

The core muscles work as stabilizers for the entire body and help the body function more effectively by working together to supply strength and coordinated movement.

Do each exercise for 20 seconds. Rest 30 seconds after each round.

EXERCISE	WORK	REST
V-Up	0:20	—
Double-Cross Reach	0:20	—
Russian Twist	0:20	—
↻ REPEAT 8 ROUNDS		REST 30 SECONDS

 CAUTION

Strengthening your core has many benefits, but like any other muscle group, the muscles that comprise your core need rest and recovery. Try to avoid back-to-back workouts that isolate your core muscles.

TOTAL TIME 10:00 BOOTY BLAST

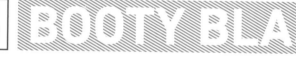

Blast your butt, hamstrings, and quads in this intense lower-body routine that also engages the core and incorporates pelvis stability and balance.

Do each exercise for 30 seconds. Rest 30 seconds after each round.

EXERCISE	WORK	REST
Pigeon Peel	0:30	—
Butterfly Peel	0:30	—
Lateral Lift	0:30	—
Pedal	0:30	—
↻ REPEAT 4 ROUNDS		REST 30 SECONDS

TOTAL TIME
19:55

METABOLIC MAYHEM

Metabolism is the process by which your body converts food into energy. This workout is all about boosting your metabolism to burn more calories. Multiple fast-paced, compound exercises performed back-to-back will ignite your body's fat-burning furnace.

Do all three rounds following the specified work-to-rest ratio. Rest one minute after each round.

EXERCISE	ROUND 1		ROUND 2		ROUND 3	
	WORK	REST	WORK	REST	WORK	REST
Squat Jump	0:30	0:30	0:30	0:15	0:30	0:10
Sprint	0:30	0:30	0:30	0:15	0:30	0:10
Pedal	0:30	0:30	0:30	0:15	0:30	0:10
Shoulder Press	0:30	0:30	0:30	0:15	0:30	0:10
Cross-Country Seal	0:30	0:30	0:30	0:15	0:30	0:10
Burpee	0:30	0:30	0:30	0:15	0:30	0:10
X-Jack	0:30	0:30	0:30	0:15	0:30	0:10
	REST 1 MINUTE		REST 1 MINUTE		REST 1 MINUTE	

TOTAL TIME
7:30

SPRINT FOR HIIT

Sprinting is arguably one of the most challenging forms of exercise. It requires you to run as hard as you can, focusing all your energy and power into short, intense bursts. The benefits of sprinting are worth the effort, as it raises your anaerobic threshold and obliterates calories in the process.

Do each exercise for 30 seconds. Rest 30 seconds after each round.

EXERCISE	WORK	REST
Sprint	0:30	—
Mountain Climber	0:30	—
Sprint	0:30	—
Diagonal Mountain Climber	0:30	—
⟳ REPEAT 3 ROUNDS		REST 30 SECONDS

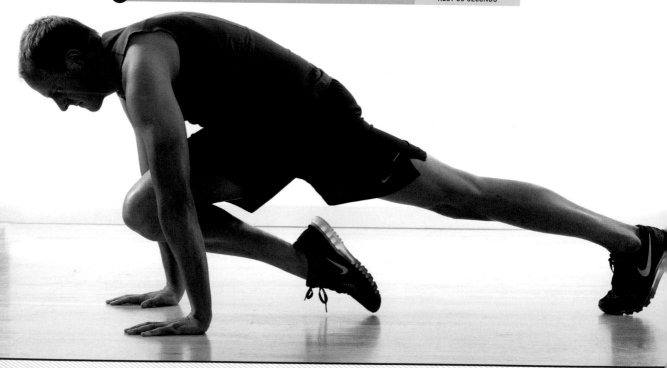

TOTAL BODY BURN

TOTAL TIME
22:30

This routine combines explosive cardio elements, like sprinting, with large muscle compound exercises, such as squat jumps and military push-ups.

Do each exercise for 30 seconds. Do three rounds of each set before moving to the next. Rest 30 seconds after each round.

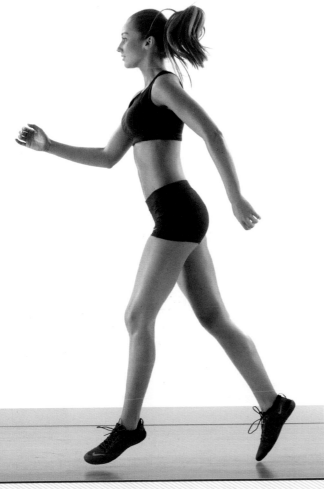

EXERCISE	WORK	REST
Sprint	0:30	—
Pedal	0:30	—
Cross-Country Seal	0:30	—
Squat Jump	0:30	—
⟳ REPEAT 3 ROUNDS		REST 30 SECONDS

EXERCISE	WORK	REST
Burpee	0:30	—
T-Stand Kick (right)	0:30	—
Military Push-Up	0:30	—
T-Stand Kick (left)	0:30	—
⟳ REPEAT 3 ROUNDS		REST 30 SECONDS

EXERCISE	WORK	REST
High Knees	0:30	—
Side Push-Up (right)	0:30	—
Squat Thrust	0:30	—
Side Push-Up (left)	0:30	—
⟳ REPEAT 3 ROUNDS		REST 30 SECONDS

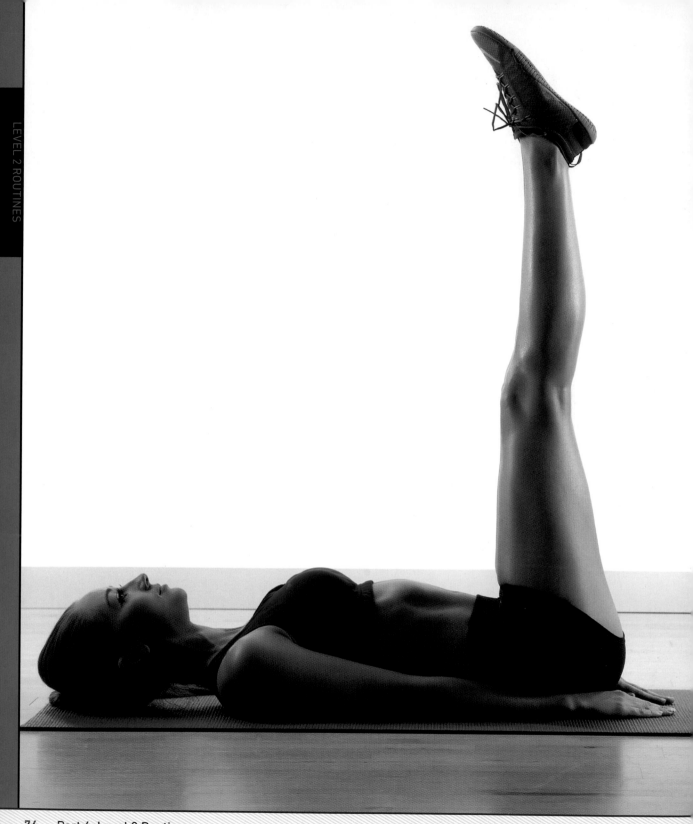

TOTAL TIME 30:00 PLYO-CARDIO

This multi-level routine couples intense cardiovascular exercises from Level 1 with plyometrics from Level 2 to create an incredibly challenging total-body workout. At a 4:1 work-to-rest ratio, this routine is relentless. Focus on your form, but push as hard as you can.

Do each exercise for 30 seconds. Do three rounds of each set before moving to the next. Rest 30 seconds after each round.

SET 1

EXERCISE	WORK	REST
Sprint	0:30	—
X-Jack	0:30	—
Cross-Country Seal	0:30	—
Mountain Climber	0:30	—
REPEAT 3 ROUNDS		REST 30 SECONDS

SET 2

EXERCISE	WORK	REST
Squat	0:30	—
Reverse Lunge	0:30	—
Squat Jump	0:30	—
Pedal	0:30	—
REPEAT 3 ROUNDS		REST 30 SECONDS

SET 3

EXERCISE	WORK	REST
Military Push-Up	0:30	—
High Knees	0:30	—
Diagonal Mountain Climber	0:30	—
Tuck Jump	0:30	—
REPEAT 3 ROUNDS		REST 30 SECONDS

SET 4

EXERCISE	WORK	REST
Jumping Jack	0:30	—
V-Up	0:30	—
Pike	0:30	—
Double-Cross Reach	0:30	—
REPEAT 3 ROUNDS		REST 30 SECONDS

MAXIMUS

TOTAL TIME 14:00

Bump it up a notch with eight total-body exercises engineered to firm and burn. Push as hard as possible; maximal effort equals maximal results.

Do each exercise for 30 seconds, followed by a 15-second rest. Rest one minute after each round.

EXERCISE	WORK	REST
X-Jack	0:30	0:15
Spiderman	0:30	0:15
Squat Jump	0:30	0:15
Pedal	0:30	0:15
Shoulder Press	0:30	0:15
Lateral Lift	0:30	0:15
V-Up	0:30	0:15
Double-Cross Reach	0:30	0:15

 REPEAT 2 ROUNDS — REST 1 MINUTE

HIIT-MAN

TOTAL TIME 7:30

This workout pushes your body to the limit with a series of "killer" exercises targeting your entire body by combining plyometric, strength-training, and cardio movements.

Do each exercise for 30 seconds. Rest 30 seconds after each round.

EXERCISE	WORK	REST
Tuck Jump	0:30	0:00
Diagonal Mountain Climber	0:30	0:00
Burpee	0:30	0:00
Spiderman	0:30	0:00

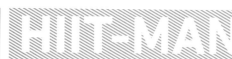 **REPEAT 3 ROUNDS** — REST 30 SECONDS

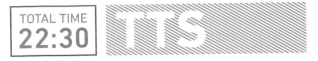

TOTAL TIME
22:30

TTS

Tone, tighten, and strengthen with three sets of high-intensity exercises. This routine will keep you on your toes.

Do each exercise for 30 seconds. Do three rounds of each set before moving to the next. Rest 30 seconds after each round.

SET 1

EXERCISE	WORK	REST
Cross-Country Seal	0:30	—
Squat Jump	0:30	—
X-Jack	0:30	—
Pedal	0:30	—
⟳ REPEAT 3 TIMES	REST 30 SECONDS	

SET 2

EXERCISE	WORK	REST
Grasshopper	0:30	—
T-Stand Kick (right)	0:30	—
Burpee	0:30	—
T-Stand Kick (left)	0:30	—
⟳ REPEAT 3 TIMES	REST 30 SECONDS	

SET 3

EXERCISE	WORK	REST
V-Up	0:30	—
Push-Up	0:30	—
Russian Twist	0:30	—
In-and-Out Abs	0:30	—
⟳ REPEAT 3 TIMES	REST 30 SECONDS	

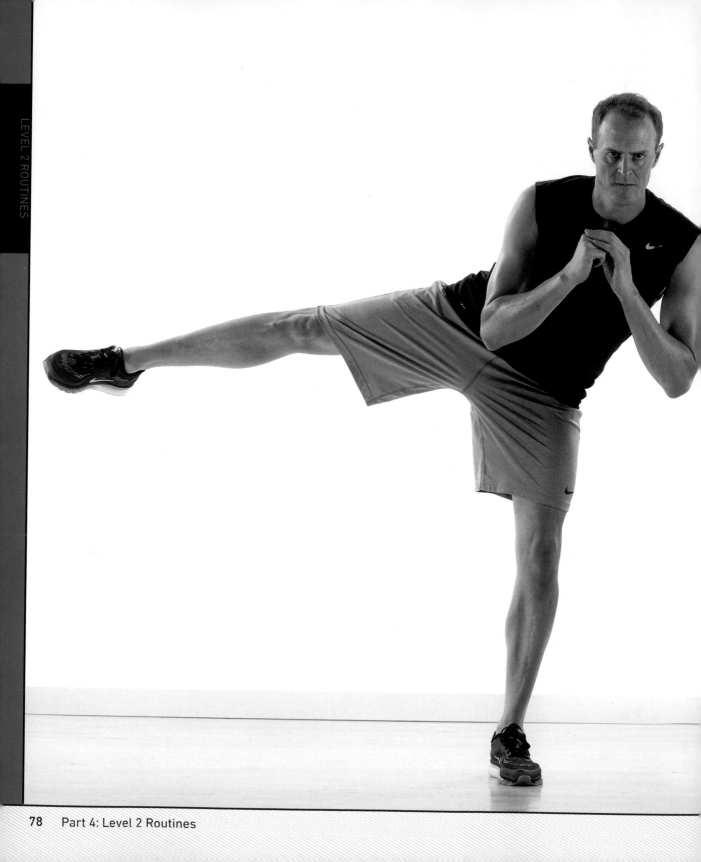

BANISH FAT

TOTAL TIME
30:00

HIIT is an efficient way to burn body fat, especially the visceral fat around the core, which has been linked with cardiovascular disease and type 2 diabetes. So pick up the pace and push as hard as you can!

Do each exercise for 30 seconds. Do three rounds of each set before moving to the next. Rest 30 seconds after each round.

TRAINER TIP

In Set 2, alternate each round among the pelvic peel, the pigeon peel, and the butterfly peel.

SET 1

EXERCISE	WORK	REST
Burpee	0:30	—
Tuck Jump	0:30	—
Cross-Country Seal	0:30	—
X-Jack	0:30	—
REPEAT 3 ROUNDS		REST 30 SECONDS

SET 2

EXERCISE	WORK	REST
Squat Jump	0:30	—
Pedal	0:30	—
Lateral Lift	0:30	—
Pelvic/Pigeon/Butterfly Peel	0:30	—
REPEAT 3 ROUNDS		REST 30 SECONDS

SET 3

EXERCISE	WORK	REST
Military Push-Up	0:30	—
High Knees	0:30	—
Diagonal Mountain Climber	0:30	—
In-and-Out Abs	0:30	—
REPEAT 3 ROUNDS		REST 30 SECONDS

SET 4

EXERCISE	WORK	REST
Side Push-Up (right)	0:30	—
V-Up	0:30	—
Side Push-Up (left)	0:30	—
Double-Cross Reach	0:30	—
REPEAT 3 ROUNDS		REST 30 SECONDS

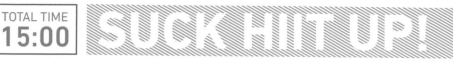

SUCK HIIT UP!

TOTAL TIME 15:00

EXERCISE	WORK	REST
Burpee	0:30	—
Diagonal Mountain Climber	0:30	—
Pedal	0:30	—
Military Push-Up	0:30	—
⟳ REPEAT 2 ROUNDS		REST 30 SECONDS

You have two choices; suck it in or suck it up! This 15-minute, total-body toner will elevate your heart rate, incinerate fat, and build both strength and confidence, so you won't ever have to suck it in again.

Do each exercise for 30 seconds. Do two rounds of each set before moving on to the next. Rest 30 seconds after each round.

EXERCISE	WORK	REST
Sprint	0:30	—
Mountain Climber	0:30	—
Squat Jump	0:30	—
Push-Up	0:30	—
⟳ REPEAT 2 ROUNDS		REST 30 SECONDS

EXERCISE	WORK	REST
Tuck Jump	0:30	—
In-and-Out Abs	0:30	—
Lateral Lunge	0:30	—
Spiderman	0:30	—
⟳ REPEAT 2 ROUNDS		REST 30 SECONDS

TRAIN INSANE

TOTAL TIME 10:00

Huge multi-muscle compound exercises meet heart-hammering, high-output cardio in this intense routine.

Do each exercise for 20 seconds, followed by a 20-second rest. Rest 30 seconds after each round.

EXERCISE	WORK	REST
Tuck Jump	0:20	0:10
Burpee	0:20	0:10
Sprint	0:20	0:10
⟳ REPEAT 5 ROUNDS		REST 30 SECONDS

TOTAL TIME
37:30

This routine brings together the very best cardiovascular exercises from Levels 1 and 2 for a heart-pounding, high-intensity workout.

Do each exercise for 30 seconds. Do five rounds of each set before moving to the next. Rest 30 seconds after each round.

EXERCISE	WORK	REST
Sprint	0:30	—
High Knees	0:30	—
Mountain Climber	0:30	—
Jumping Jack	0:30	—
REPEAT 5 ROUNDS		REST 30 SECONDS

EXERCISE	WORK	REST
Burpee	0:30	—
Cross-Country Seal	0:30	—
X-Jack	0:30	—
Grasshopper	0:30	—
REPEAT 5 ROUNDS		REST 30 SECONDS

EXERCISE	WORK	REST
Tuck Jump	0:30	—
Squat Thrust	0:30	—
Diagonal Mountain Climber	0:30	—
Sprint	0:30	—
REPEAT 5 ROUNDS		REST 30 SECONDS

TOTAL TIME
10:00

SUPERHERO CIRCUIT

This short circuit may not give you super powers, but it will help to tone and define your muscles. Move as fast as you can while maintaining proper form.

Do each exercise for 30 seconds. Rest 30 seconds between rounds.

EXERCISE	WORK	REST
Burpee	0:30	—
Spiderman	0:30	—
Squat Jump	0:30	—
Pedal	0:30	—
↻ REPEAT 4 ROUNDS		REST 30 SECONDS

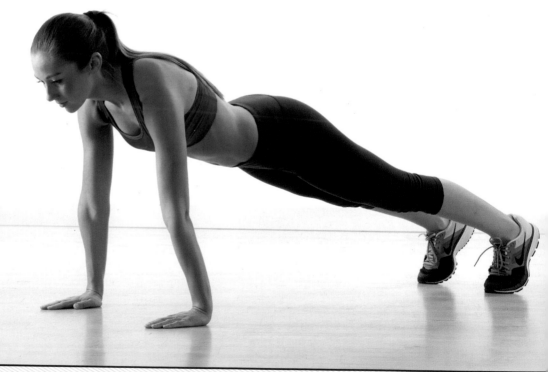

The tuck jump is as tough as it gets, but worth the effort. Tuck jumps incinerate calories, improve athletic performance, and have been shown to improve bone density.

Do as many tuck jumps as possible during each interval, followed by the specified rest. Rest 30 seconds after each round.

TOTAL TIME
9:00

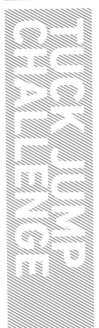

TUCK JUMP CHALLENGE

TRAINER TIP

If necessary, pause between the jumps, sink into the squat position and "set" yourself between each jump. This will decrease the frequency of the jumps and allow greater recovery time as you build your stamina.

EXERCISE	WORK	REST
Tuck Jump	0:30	0:15
Tuck Jump	0:30	0:30
Tuck Jump	0:30	0:15
⟳ REPEAT 3 ROUNDS	REST 30 SECONDS	

TOTAL TIME 10:00 TOUGH LOVE

Getting the most out of HIIT requires commitment and dedication. Be tough on yourself and accept only 100 percent effort. This routine features Level 1 exercises in set 1 and Level 2 exercises in set 2. Feel the difference and see how far you've come toward achieving your goals.

Do each exercise for 30 seconds. Do two rounds of each set before moving to the next. Rest 30 seconds between rounds.

EXERCISE	WORK	REST
Sprint	0:30	—
High Knees	0:30	—
Mountain Climber	0:30	—
Jumping Jack	0:30	—
⟳ REPEAT 2 ROUNDS		REST 30 SECONDS

EXERCISE	WORK	REST
Cross-Country Seal	0:30	—
Tuck Jump	0:30	—
Grasshopper	0:30	—
X-Jack	0:30	—
⟳ REPEAT 2 ROUNDS		REST 30 SECONDS

TOTAL TIME 10:00 PUSH It

This routine also includes some Level 1 exercises. If you've been working hard, these should be much easier than they were when you started. Hard work, dedication, and sweat will get you where you want to be.

Do each exercise for 30 seconds. Do two rounds of each set before moving to the next. Rest 30 seconds between rounds.

EXERCISE	WORK	REST
Squat Thrust	0:30	—
Squat	0:30	—
Kneeling Push-Up	0:30	—
Pike	0:30	—
REPEAT 2 ROUNDS		REST 30 SECONDS

EXERCISE	WORK	REST
Burpee	0:30	—
Squat Jump	0:30	
Push-Up	0:30	—
V-Up	0:30	—
REPEAT 2 ROUNDS		REST 30 SECONDS

ARMORED ABS

This core-focused routine targets your abs as well as your hip flexors, lower back, and legs, creating a toned, tighter, stronger, and more stable midsection.

Do each exercise for 30 seconds. Do three rounds of each set before moving to the next. Rest 30 seconds after each round.

SET 1

EXERCISE	WORK	REST
V-Up	0:30	0:00
Side Plank (right)	0:30	0:00
Plank	0:30	0:00
Side Plank (left)	0:30	0:00
REPEAT 3 ROUNDS		REST 30 SECONDS

SET 2

EXERCISE	WORK	REST
Diagonal Mountain Climber	0:30	0:00
Double-Cross Reach	0:30	0:00
Russian Twist	0:30	0:00
In-and-Out Abs	0:30	0:00
REPEAT 3 ROUNDS		REST 30 SECONDS

SET 3

EXERCISE	WORK	REST
Pike	0:30	0:00
Circles (right)	0:30	0:00
Circles (left)	0:30	0:00
Bicycle Crunch	0:30	0:00
REPEAT 3 ROUNDS		REST 30 SECONDS

QUAD KILLER

TOTAL TIME 10:00

Ten pounds of muscle will burn 50 calories in a day spent at rest, while 10 pounds of fat will burn only 20 calories. Now imagine how many calories lean muscle will burn while working! The quads are some of the largest muscles in the body and therefore consume the most calories both at work and rest.

Do each exercise for 30 seconds, followed by a 10-second rest. Rest 30 seconds after each round.

EXERCISE	WORK	REST
Squat	0:30	0:10
Pedal	0:30	0:10
Squat Jump	0:30	0:10
REPEAT 4 ROUNDS		REST 30 SECONDS

PEEL OUT

TOTAL TIME 10:00

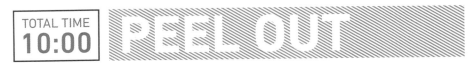

The pelvic peel is a simple exercise, but very effective for maintaining strength in the lower back and preventing lower-back pain. Pelvic bridging also strengthens the paraspinal muscles, the quads, hamstrings, abdominals, and the glutes. The pigeon and butterfly variations add intensity to the routine.

Do each exercise for 30 seconds, followed by a 10-second rest. Rest 30 seconds after each round.

EXERCISE	WORK	REST
Pelvic Peel	0:30	0:10
Pigeon Peel	0:30	0:10
Butterfly Peel	0:30	0:10
REPEAT 4 ROUNDS		REST 30 SECONDS

 TRAINER TIP

Focus on engaging the glutes as you lift your hips during the pelvic peel. For an added challenge, try doing any of the peels with your feet elevated on a bench or BOSU ball.

MAKE HIIT BURN

There's nothing more satisfying than feeling that deep burn in your muscles as you fight for one extra rep, an inch more depth, or five seconds more work. Push yourself and feel the burn!

Do each exercise for 30 seconds. Do two rounds of each set. Rest 30 seconds after each round.

SET 1

EXERCISE	WORK	REST
Cross-Country Seal	0:30	—
X-Jack	0:30	—
Burpee	0:30	—
Tuck Jump	0:30	—
REPEAT 2 ROUNDS		REST 30 SECONDS

SET 2

EXERCISE	WORK	REST
Squat	0:30	—
Reverse Lunge	0:30	—
Squat Jump	0:30	—
Pedal	0:30	—
REPEAT 2 ROUNDS		REST 30 SECONDS

SET 3

EXERCISE	WORK	REST
Push-Up	0:30	—
Double-Cross Reach	0:30	—
Diagonal Mountain Climber	0:30	—
V-Up	0:30	—
REPEAT 2 ROUNDS		REST 30 SECONDS

KILLING HIIT

TOTAL TIME 18:00

HIIT workouts are tough, but don't let that stop you. This routine keeps things interesting with exercises that challenge every part of your body.

Do each exercise for 20 seconds, followed by a 10-second rest. Rest one minute after each round.

EXERCISE	WORK	REST
Sprint	0:20	0:10
Pedal	0:20	0:10
High Knees	0:20	0:10
Push-Up	0:20	0:10
V-Up	0:20	0:10
Tuck Jump	0:20	0:10
Squat Jump	0:20	0:10
Grasshopper	0:20	0:10
Triceps Dip	0:20	0:10
Russian Twist	0:20	0:10
REPEAT 3 ROUNDS	**REST 1 MINUTE**	

TOTAL TIME 12:00

THE BEAST

This routine pairs traditional strength-training exercises with explosive plyometric and cardio movements for a workout challenge that will bring out your wild side.

Do each exercise for 20 seconds, followed by a 10-second rest. Rest one minute after each round.

EXERCISE	WORK	REST
Burpee	0:20	0:10
Side Push-Up (right)	0:20	0:10
Tuck Jump	0:20	0:10
Side Push-Up (left)	0:20	0:10
Sprint	0:20	0:10
Spiderman	0:20	0:10
↻ REPEAT 3 ROUNDS		REST 1 MINUTE

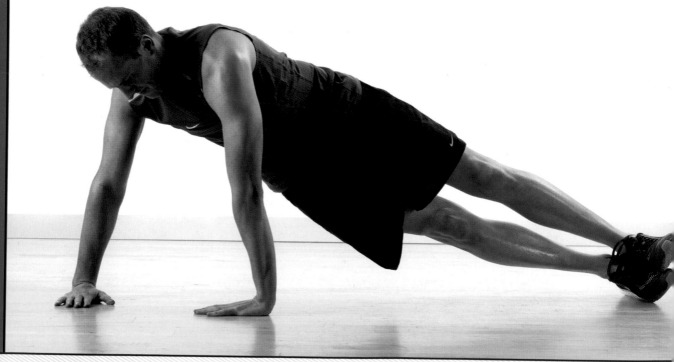

TOTAL TIME
12:00

YOU CAN DO HIIT!

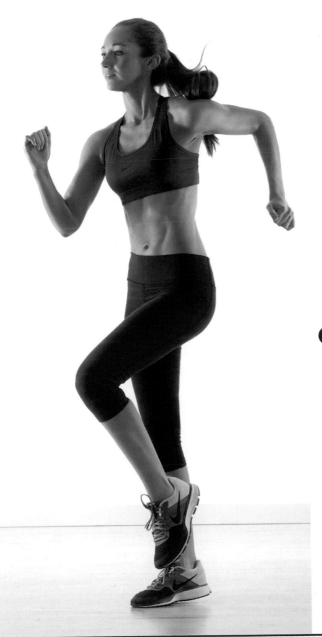

If you can make it through eight rounds of this routine then you truly can do HIIT. Take pride in the progress you've made, but keep pushing. Level 3 is up next!

Do each exercise for 20 seconds. Rest 30 seconds after each round.

EXERCISE	WORK	REST
Sprint	0:20	—
Burpee	0:20	—
Diagonal Mountain Climber	0:20	—
⟳ **REPEAT 8 ROUNDS**		**REST 30 SECONDS**

Committing to HIIT for just three days will make it easier to incorporate it as part of your regular lifestyle. Each head-to-toe workout combines high-output cardio and compound strength exercises to give you a firm foundation for HIIT.

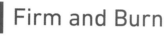

DAY	ROUTINE
1	Firm and Burn
2	Train Insane
3	Banish Fat

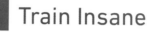

TRAINER TIPS

- To decrease the risk of injury and prepare yourself to perform at 100 percent, remember to warm up each day before beginning your HIIT routine.

- Focus on form before speed. Make sure you know how to do each exercise properly before beginning your routine.

- Stay hydrated and don't let your diet undo all your hard work! To get the results you want, you'll need to work hard and watch your caloric intake.

The 7-Day Challenge introduces some new HIIT routine formats and features exercises designed to burn fat, lose weight, increase strength, and improve athletic performance. Give it all you've got, and you'll be amazed at the results you can achieve in just one week.

DAY	ROUTINE
1	Fit Frenzy
2	Peel Out
3	Maximus
4	Metabolic Mayhem
5	Armored Abs
6	Push It
7	Ready to Sweat

TRAINER TIPS

- To perform your best and prevent injury, begin each routine with a three- to five-minute warm up.

- The 7-Day Challenge introduces more athletic exercises, so form is more important than ever. Be sure you know how to do each exercise correctly before beginning your routine.

- Expect to be sore. If your workouts are as intense as they should be, you will be sore the next day. Remember that sore muscles are not the same as pain due to injury.

- This program was designed to be undertaken on back-to-back days, but if necessary, you can take a rest day between workouts. Listen to your body and allow the appropriate recovery time.

If you're willing to commit to two weeks of HIIT, you'll be able to see a change in your body. The routines in this program will help you lose weight, build strength, and improve cardiovascular endurance with a combination of body weight and plyometric exercises. The 14-Day Challenge incorporates focused routines for the core and lower body to break up the high-impact routines and ensure you can give 100 percent each and every day.

DAY	ROUTINE
1	You Can Do HIIT
2	The Beast
3	Fit Frenzy
4	Tough Love
5	Suck HIIT Up!
6	Banish Fat
7	Train Insane

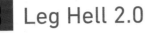
LEVEL 2 ROUTINES

8 Leg Hell 2.0

9 Plyo-Cardio

10 Maximus

11 Killing HIIT

12 Firm and Burn

13 Make HIIT Burn

14 Ready to Sweat

TRAINER TIPS

- Make sure you warm up thoroughly before undertaking any of the routines in this challenge.

- Remember that quality is more important than quantity. The 14-Day Challenge introduces more athletic exercises, which means attention to form is critical.

- Stay mentally strong and focus on your goals. Two weeks takes dedication. It's easy for "just one day off" to turn into two and then three. Stick with it.

- Be aware of what you eat. You'll see greater changes if you are disciplined in your eating as well as your exercise.

If you want to get results from HIIT, you have to make it a regular part of your schedule. After four weeks of intense workouts, you'll be strong and confident enough to tackle Level 3. Stick to the workout plan and reassess your fitness at the end.

DAY	ROUTINE	DAY	ROUTINE
1	Total Body Burn	8	Train Insane
2	Leg Hell 2.0	9	Hi-Low
3	Sprint for HIIT	10	Double Cross
4	Push It	11	Superhero Circuit
5	Tough Love	12	Tuck Jump Challenge
6	Suck HIIT Up!	13	Peel Out
7	Firm and Burn	14	Fit Frenzy

DAY	ROUTINE	DAY	ROUTINE
15	HIIT-Man	22	The Beast
16	Armored Abs	23	You Can Do HIIT!
17	Maximus	24	Metabolic Mayhem
18	TTS	25	Banish Fat
19	Hard Core	26	No Excuses
20	Booty Blast	27	Quad Killer
21	Plyo-Cardio	28	Addicted to Sweat

TRAINER TIPS

- To perform your best and prevent injury, begin each routine with a thorough warm up.

- Setting aside a specific time for HIIT each day will make it easier to stay on track. Make a plan each week for your workouts and stick to it.

- You will likely experience soreness if you haven't been working out regularly, especially during the first week. Take time to stretch and use a foam roller to aid in muscle recovery.

- If you're making the commitment to do HIIT for 28 days, commit to monitoring your diet as well. Getting the results you want takes discipline.

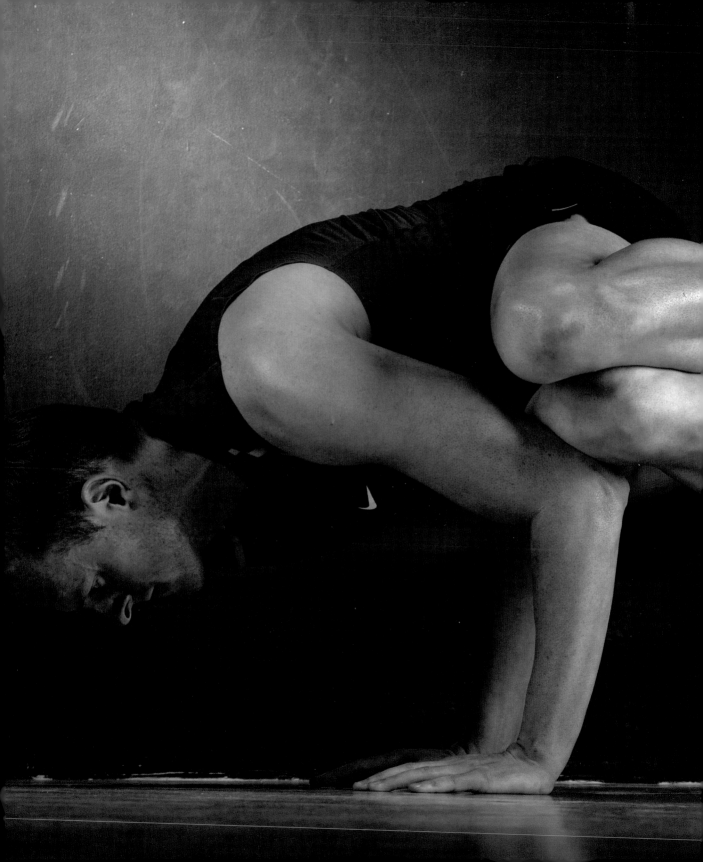

The Level 3 routines are as tough as it gets. They comprise the ultimate HIIT challenge, fusing high-output cardio with large-muscle compound exercises and plyometrics to provide a workout like no other.

The routines in this part range from a few minutes to an hour and include a variety of work-to-rest ratios to keep your body in a state of confusion for maximum results. Many of the routines in Level 3 involve dynamic balance and multiplanar motions to challenge your core stability and athletic ability.

LEVEL UP

This routine features one exercise from each of the three difficulty levels in this book. Each exercise will increase your heart rate, challenge your strength, and incinerate calories.

Do each exercise for 30 seconds. Rest 30 seconds after each round.

EXERCISE	TIME OR REPS	REST
Sprint	0:30	—
Diagonal Mountain Climber	0:30	—
Tuck Jump Burpee	0:30	—
⟳ **REPEAT 8 ROUNDS**		**REST 30 SECONDS**

TRAINER TIP

When sprinting, try to drive with the arms as this will help to power the legs. Relax your hands and jaw and keep a slight forward lean to the body with core engaged.

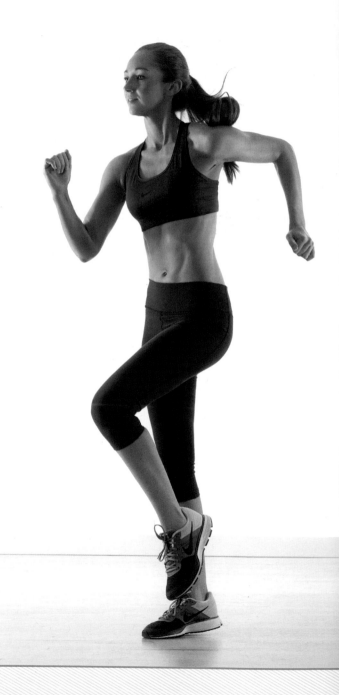

HIGH FIVE

Five exercises, five minutes of work, five rounds! If you survive this routine you deserve a high five ... although you may not be able to lift your arm to receive it!

Do each exercise for one minute. Rest one minute after each round.

EXERCISE	WORK	REST
Single Leg Burpee	1:00	—
Squat Pedal	1:00	—
Plyo Trio	1:00	—
Star	1:00	—
Sprinter Sit-Up	1:00	—
⟳ **REPEAT 5 ROUNDS**		REST 1 MINUTE

TRAINER TIP

It's extremely challenging to do the plyo trio for a full minute. If you feel your form suffering, drop to your knees and continue.

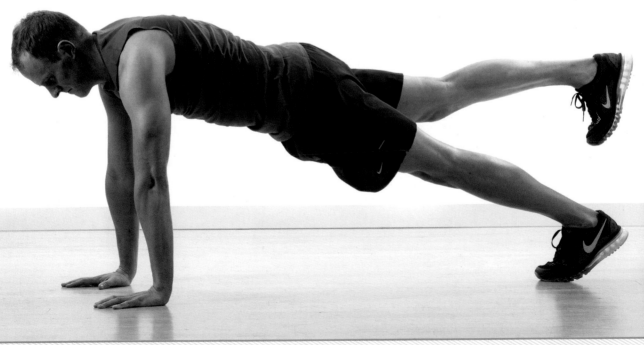

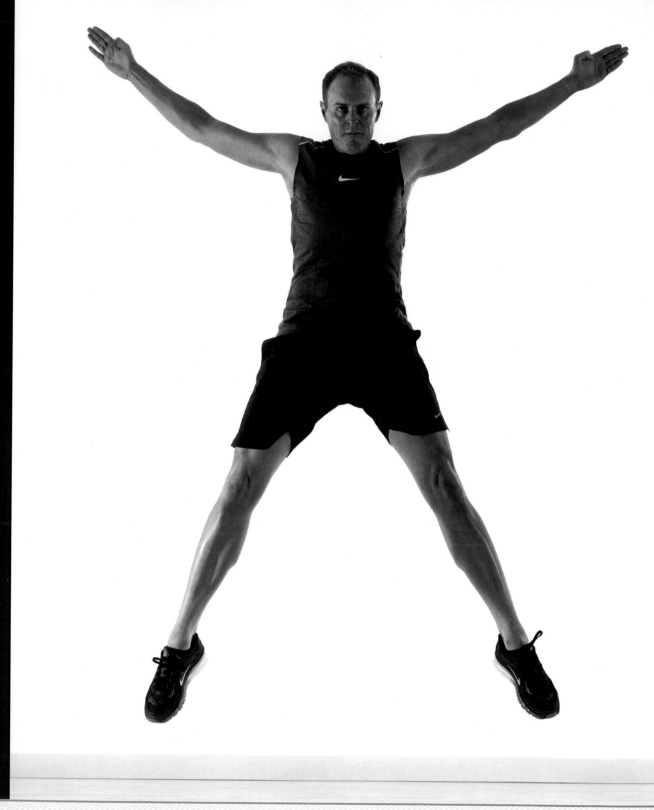

TOTAL TIME 15:00 — HARD CHARGER

A relentless drive and commitment to excellence are required for this routine. Back-to-back high-tempo, compound exercises combine with plyometrics and traditional cardio for an incredible challenge.

Do each exercise for 30 seconds. Do three rounds of each set. Rest 30 seconds after each round.

SET 1 EXERCISE	WORK	REST
Sprint	0:30	—
Single Leg Burpee	0:30	—
Plus Jump	0:30	—
Star	0:30	—
REPEAT 3 ROUNDS		REST 30 SECONDS

SET 2 EXERCISE	WORK	REST
Squat Pedal	0:30	—
In and Outs	0:30	—
Skater Jump	0:30	—
Reverse Push-Up	0:30	—
REPEAT 3 ROUNDS		REST 30 SECONDS

TOTAL TIME 9:00 — FULL THROTTLE

Get ready to push yourself to the max with this plyometric-focused routine. Keep your movements fast and explosive.

Do each exercise for 30 seconds. Rest 30 seconds after each round.

EXERCISE	WORK	REST
Single Leg Burpee	0:30	—
Plus Jumps	0:30	—
Tuck Jump Burpee	0:30	—
Lizard Hops	0:30	—
Star	0:30	—
REPEAT 3 ROUNDS		REST 30 SECONDS

POWER HOUR 1

The appeal of most HIIT routines is that they're over quickly, but they don't have to be. If you're ready to take on a full hour of HIIT, this is for you. Do 10 minutes of dynamic stretching before beginning the cardio warm-up.

WARM UP
5:00

WARM-UP

Before you give it all you've got for the main workout, get your heart pumping with a quick cardio warm-up. Start off nice and easy; you don't need to push yourself to the max yet.

EXERCISE	WORK	REST
Sprint	0:30	—
Jumping Jack	0:30	—
Lateral Lunge	0:30	—
High Knees	0:30	—
Squat	0:30	—
REPEAT 2 ROUNDS		NO REST BETWEEN ROUNDS

WORKOUT
45:00

WORKOUT

This is the main event. Push yourself as hard as possible for 45 minutes of fat-burning, strength-building, muscle-toning work.

Do each exercise for 30 seconds. Do three rounds of each set. Rest 30 seconds after each round.

SET 1		
EXERCISE	WORK	REST
Sprint	0:30	—
Cross-Country Seal	0:30	—
Mountain Climber	0:30	—
Skater Jump	0:30	—
REPEAT 3 ROUNDS		REST 30 SECONDS

SET 2

EXERCISE	WORK	REST
Tuck Jump Burpee	0:30	—
Plus Jump	0:30	—
Diagonal Mountain Climber	0:30	—
Star	0:30	—
REPEAT 3 ROUNDS		REST 30 SECONDS

SET 3

EXERCISE	WORK	REST
Squat	0:30	—
Reverse Lunge	0:30	—
Squat Jump	0:30	—
Pedal	0:30	—
REPEAT 3 ROUNDS		REST 30 SECONDS

SET 4

EXERCISE	WORK	REST
Single Leg Burpee	0:30	—
Grasshopper	0:30	—
Log Hop T-Stand	0:30	—
Dragon Walk	0:30	—
REPEAT 3 ROUNDS		REST 30 SECONDS

SET 5

EXERCISE	WORK	REST
Squat Pedal	0:30	—
Lizard Hop	0:30	—
In and Outs	0:30	—
Plyo Push-Up	0:30	—
REPEAT 3 ROUNDS		REST 30 SECONDS

SET 6

EXERCISE	WORK	REST
1-2 Push	0:30	—
Flutter-Up	0:30	—
V-Up Doubles	0:30	—
Sprinter Sit-Up	0:30	—
REPEAT 3 ROUNDS		REST 30 SECONDS

TRAINER TIP

If you're struggling, increase the rest time to one minute after each round.

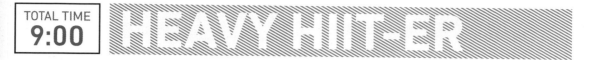

TOTAL TIME 9:00 — HEAVY HIIT-ER

This challenging total-body routine includes plyometric, multiplanar, and dynamic stability exercises to push you to your limits.

Do each exercise for 30 seconds. Do three rounds of each set before moving to the next. Rest 30 seconds after each round.

SET 1

EXERCISE	WORK	REST
Single Leg Burpee	0:30	—
Star	0:30	—
Lizard Hop	0:30	—
Tuck Jump Burpee	0:30	—
⟳ REPEAT 3 ROUNDS	REST 30 SECONDS	

SET 2

EXERCISE	WORK	REST
Squat Pedal	0:30	—
Skater Jump	0:30	—
In and Outs	0:30	—
Log Hop T-Stand	0:30	—
⟳ REPEAT 3 ROUNDS	REST 30 SECONDS	

SET 3

EXERCISE	WORK	REST
1-2-Push	0:30	—
Sprinter Sit-Up	0:30	—
Flutter-Up	0:30	—
Up and Overs	0:30	—
⟳ REPEAT 3 ROUNDS	REST 30 SECONDS	

LEG HELL 3.0

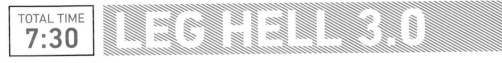

Your large lower-body muscles will be put to the test with this quad-killing routine.

Do each exercise for 30 seconds. Rest 30 seconds after each round.

EXERCISE	WORK	REST
Squat Pedal	0:30	—
In and Outs	0:30	—
Squat Jump	0:30	—
Pedal	0:30	—
↻ REPEAT 3 ROUNDS	REST 30 SECONDS	

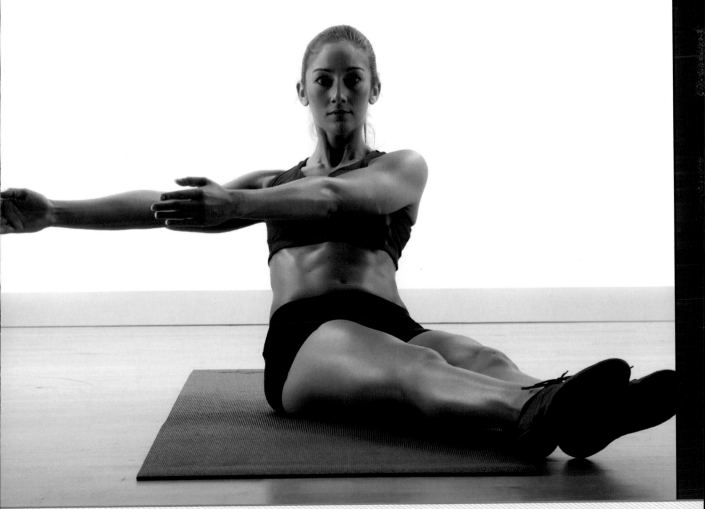

TOTAL TIME
60:00

POWER HOUR 2

Who said you need to keep it short and sweet? Prepare to burn over 800 calories with this grueling, hour-long workout. Be sure to do 10 minutes of dynamic stretching before beginning the cardio warm-up.

WARM UP
5:00

WARM-UP

Start things off with a quick cardio warm-up. Don't push yourself yet; you should be working at 50 to 75 percent of your power.

EXERCISE	WORK	REST
Sprint	0:30	—
Jumping Jack	0:30	—
High Knees	0:30	—
X-Jack	0:30	—
Squat	0:30	—
⟳ REPEAT 2 ROUNDS		NO REST BETWEEN ROUNDS

WORKOUT
45:00

WORKOUT

Now it's time to kick it into high gear. Dig deep and keep your goals in mind.

Do each exercise for 30 seconds. Do three rounds of each set. Rest 30 seconds after each round.

SET 1		
EXERCISE	WORK	REST
High Knees	0:30	—
1-2 Push	0:30	—
Tuck Jump Burpee	0:30	—
Jumping Jack	0:30	—
⟳ REPEAT 3 ROUNDS		REST 30 SECONDS

SET 2

EXERCISE	WORK	REST
Squat Pedal	0:30	—
Single Leg Burpee	0:30	—
Lateral Lunge	0:30	—
Star	0:30	—
REPEAT 3 ROUNDS		REST 30 SECONDS

SET 3

EXERCISE	WORK	REST
Squat Jump	0:30	—
Skater Jump	0:30	—
Pedal	0:30	—
Mountain Climber	0:30	—
REPEAT 3 ROUNDS		REST 30 SECONDS

SET 4

EXERCISE	WORK	REST
Diagonal Mountain Climber	0:30	—
Log Hop T-Stand	0:30	—
Sprint	0:30	—
1-2 Push	0:30	—
REPEAT 3 ROUNDS		REST 30 SECONDS

TRAINER TIP

Your mind and body are going to scream at you to stop during this workout. Remember that you get out what you put in. Push as hard as possible to get maximum results.

SET 5

EXERCISE	WORK	REST
Squat	0:30	—
Triceps Dip	0:30	—
Lizard Hop	0:30	—
Plus Jump	0:30	—
REPEAT 3 ROUNDS		REST 30 SECONDS

SET 6

EXERCISE	WORK	REST
V-Up	0:30	—
Sprinter Sit-Up	0:30	—
Russian Twist	0:30	—
Up and Overs	0:30	—
REPEAT 3 ROUNDS		REST 30 SECONDS

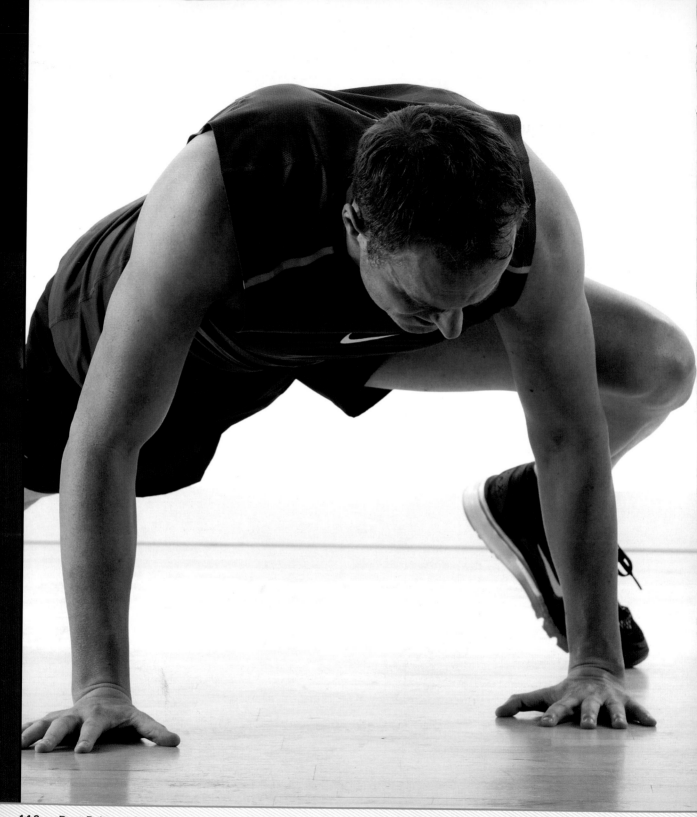

…E YOURSELF

…lders, back, abs, and legs this routine will … ith each exercise.

… rounds of each set. Rest 30 seconds after each round.

EXERCISE	WORK	REST
	0:30	—
	0:30	—
…l Lift	0:30	—
… Peel	0:30	—
…UNDS	REST 30 SECONDS	

…RK	REST
…:30	—
…:30	—
0:30	—
0:30	—
REST 30 SECONDS	

SET 3

EXERCISE	WORK	REST
Side Press (right)	0:30	—
Military Push-Up	0:30	—
Side Press (left)	0:30	—
Plank	0:30	—
REPEAT 3 ROUNDS	REST 30 SECONDS	

TOTAL TIME 15:00

CONQUER

An all-out onslaught is required to conquer this fast-paced, head-to-toe routine.

Do each exercise for 30 seconds. Do three rounds of each set. Rest 30 seconds after each round.

SET 1

EXERCISE	WORK	REST
Sprint	0:30	—
Single Leg Burpee	0:30	—
Cross-Country Seal	0:30	—
X-Jack	0:30	—
REPEAT 3 ROUNDS	REST 30 SECONDS	

SET 2

EXERCISE	WORK	REST
Dragon Walk	0:30	—
Sprinter Sit-Up	0:30	—
Reverse Push-Up	0:30	—
Up and Overs	0:30	—
REPEAT 3 ROUNDS	REST 30 SECONDS	

TOTAL TIME 12:00

POSTURE PERFECT

Doing regular posture-building exercises can pack a double punch when it comes to losing your gut. Good posture makes you look slimmer, and sticking to a posture-building routine every day will strengthen your ab muscles and help you earn your six-pack.

Do each exercise for 30 seconds. Rest 30 seconds after each round.

EXERCISE	WORK	REST
Pike	0:30	—
V-Up Double	0:30	—
Side Plank (right)	0:30	—
Sprinter Sit-Up	0:30	—
Side Plank (left)	0:30	—
Double-Cross Reach	0:30	—
Plank	0:30	—
REPEAT 3 ROUNDS	REST 30 SECONDS	

KILLER CARDIO

The saying "what doesn't kill you makes you stronger" is true of this routine. It features a killer combination of exercises from all three skill levels that will improve your strength and endurance.

Do each exercise for 30 seconds. Do three rounds of each set. Rest 30 seconds after each round.

SET 1		
EXERCISE	WORK	REST
Sprint	0:30	—
Star	0:30	—
Plus Jump	0:30	—
Cross-Country Seal	0:30	—
↻ REPEAT 3 ROUNDS		REST 30 SECONDS

SET 2		
EXERCISE	WORK	REST
High Knees	0:30	—
Single Leg Burpee	0:30	—
Lizard Hop	0:30	—
X-Jack	0:30	—
↻ REPEAT 3 ROUNDS		REST 30 SECONDS

SET 3		
EXERCISE	WORK	REST
Jumping Jack	0:30	—
Tuck Jump Burpee	0:30	—
Grasshopper	0:30	—
Mountain Climber	0:30	—
↻ REPEAT 3 ROUNDS		REST 30 SECONDS

CHALLENGE

DEFIN

Turn heads with the defined shou create. Aim for maximum reps w

Do each exercise for 30 seconds. Do three

SET 1	
EXERCISE	
Squat	
Pedal	
Latera	
Pelvic	
↻ REPEAT 3 R	

REDLINE

If yo
speed
would
the wa
this tu
cardio r
your eng

Do each exer
seconds. Rest
each round.

SET 2	
EXERCISE	
1-2 Push	0
V-Up	
Diagonal Mountain Climber	
Flutter-Up	
↻ REPEAT 3 ROUNDS	

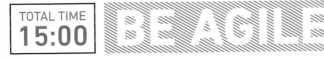

BE AGILE

This combination of exercises will challenge your balance, stabilization, and athletic performance to make you more agile on and off the field.

Do each exercise for 20 seconds. Rest 30 seconds after each round.

EXERCISE	WORK	REST
Log Hop T-Stand	0:20	—
Spiderman	0:20	—
Plus Jump	0:20	—
Grasshopper	0:20	—
Single Leg Burpee	0:20	—
Skater Jump	0:20	—
↻ REPEAT 6 ROUNDS		REST 30 SECONDS

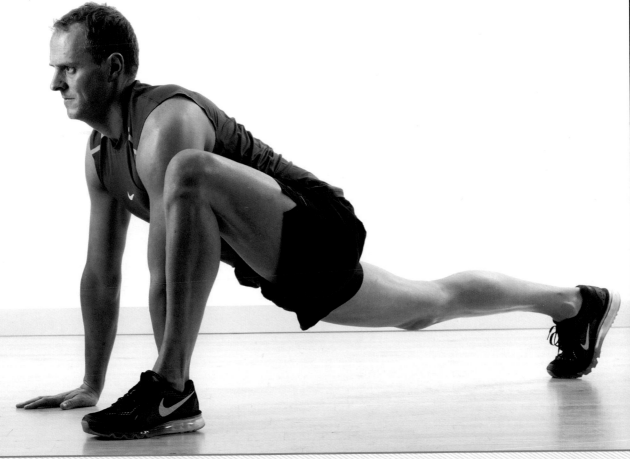

POWER HOUR 3

TOTAL TIME 60:00

If you really want to test your endurance, take on a Power Hour. Begin with 10 minutes of dynamic stretching before moving into the cardio warm-up and workout.

WARM-UP

WARM UP 5:00

After stretching, get moving with a quick cardio warm-up. Start slow; you don't need to push yourself yet.

EXERCISE	WORK	REST
Sprint	0:30	—
Jumping Jack	0:30	—
High Knees	0:30	—
X-Jack	0:30	—
Squat	0:30	—
↻ REPEAT 2 ROUNDS		NO REST BETWEEN ROUNDS

WORKOUT

WORKOUT 45:00

Push yourself as hard as you can for the next 45 minutes.

Do each exercise for 30 seconds. Do three rounds of each set. Rest 30 seconds after each round.

SET 1		
EXERCISE	WORK	REST
Cross-Country Seal	0:30	—
Shoulder Press	0:30	—
Tuck Jump Burpee	0:30	—
Squat Jump	0:30	—
↻ REPEAT 3 ROUNDS		REST 30 SECONDS

SET 2

EXERCISE	WORK	REST
Squat Pedal	0:30	—
Single Leg Burpee	0:30	—
High Knees	0:30	—
1-2 Push	0:30	—

REPEAT 3 ROUNDS   REST 30 SECONDS

SET 3

EXERCISE	WORK	REST
Log Hop T-Stand	0:30	—
Diagonal Mountain Climber	0:30	—
Grasshopper	0:30	—
X-Jack	0:30	—

REPEAT 3 ROUNDS   REST 30 SECONDS

SET 4

EXERCISE	WORK	REST
Single Leg Peel (right)	0:30	—
Single Leg Peel (left)	0:30	—
Pigeon Peel	0:30	—
Butterfly Peel	0:30	—

REPEAT 3 ROUNDS   REST 30 SECONDS

SET 5

EXERCISE	WORK	REST
Squat	0:30	—
Military Push-Up	0:30	—
Lizard Hop	0:30	—
Plus Jump	0:30	—

REPEAT 3 ROUNDS   REST 30 SECONDS

SET 6

EXERCISE	WORK	REST
V-Up	0:30	—
Sprinter Sit-Up	0:30	—
Russian Twist	0:30	—
Plank	0:30	—

REPEAT 3 ROUNDS   REST 30 SECONDS

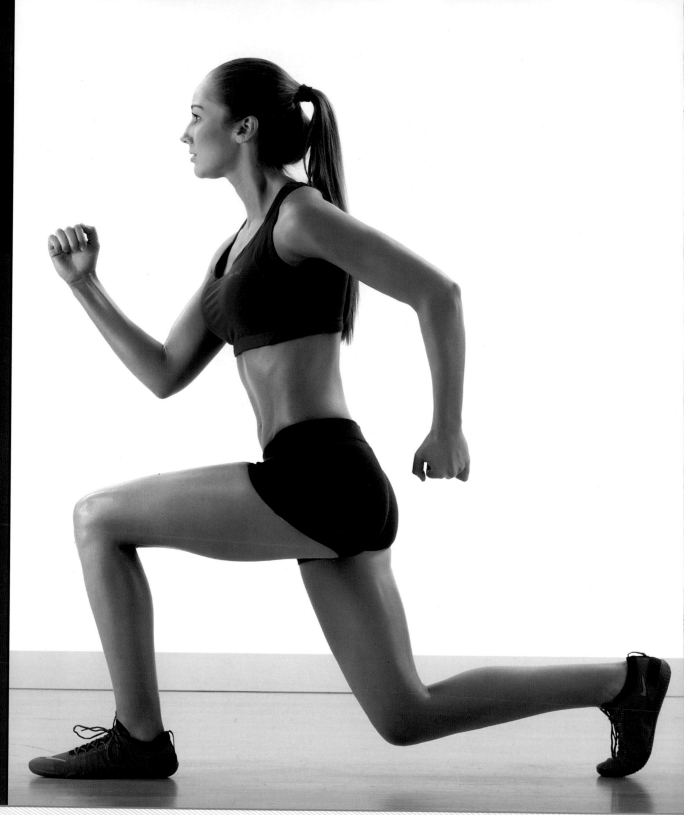

DROP SETS

TOTAL TIME 15:00

A drop set is a bodybuilding technique that allows the lifter to continue an exercise set past fatigue by moving to a lower weight, doing fewer reps, or switching to a similar exercise. This routine gives HIIT the drop set treatment, alternating plyometric exercises with their standard counterparts for incredible results.

Do each exercise for 30 seconds, followed by the specified rest. Rest 30 seconds after each round.

EXERCISE	WORK	REST
Squat Jump	0:30	—
Squat	0:30	0:30
Pedal	0:30	—
Reverse Lunge	0:30	0:30
Plyo Push-Up	0:30	—
Push-Up	0:30	0:30
REPEAT 3 ROUNDS		REST 30 SECONDS

SWEAT AND SMILE

TOTAL TIME 7:30

Push as hard as you can during this dynamic stack routine. With each round, the work-to-rest ratio increases. Sweat or regret? The choice is yours!

Do each exercise for the specified time. Complete all three rounds. Rest 30 seconds after each round.

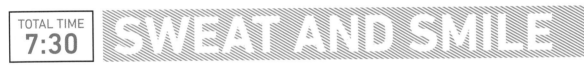

EXERCISE	ROUND 1		ROUND 2		ROUND 3	
	WORK	REST	WORK	REST	WORK	REST
Tuck Jump Burpee	0:15	0:15	0:20	0:10	0:30	—
Star	0:15	0:15	0:20	0:10	0:30	—
Lizard Hop	0:15	0:15	0:20	0:10	0:30	—
Plus Jump	0:15	0:15	0:20	0:10	0:30	—
	REST 30 SECONDS		REST 30 SECONDS		REST 30 SECONDS	

POWER HOUR 4

TOTAL TIME 60:00

Power Hour routines pull exercises from all three levels into one 60-minute, head-to-toe workout. Requiring strength, endurance, and mental toughness, these hour-long sessions are the ultimate HIIT routines! Get started with 10 minutes of dynamic stretching before the cardio warm-up.

WARM UP 5:00

WARM-UP

This quick cardio warm-up should start to raise your heart rate, but don't push too hard yet.

EXERCISE	WORK	REST
Sprint	0:30	—
Jumping Jack	0:30	—
High Knees	0:30	—
X-Jack	0:30	—
Squat	0:30	—
⟳ REPEAT 2 ROUNDS		NO REST BETWEEN ROUNDS

WORKOUT 45:00

WORKOUT

For this portion, you should be working as hard as you can. Keep moving!

Do each exercise for 30 seconds. Do three rounds of each set. Rest 30 seconds after each round.

SET 1		
EXERCISE	WORK	REST
Sprint	0:30	—
Squat	0:30	—
Shoulder Press Jack	0:30	—
Mountain Climber	0:30	—
⟳ REPEAT 3 ROUNDS		REST 30 SECONDS

SET 2

EXERCISE	WORK	REST
Burpee	0:30	—
Cros-Country Seal	0:30	—
X-Jack	0:30	—
Push-Up	0:30	—
REPEAT 3 ROUNDS		REST 30 SECONDS

SET 3

EXERCISE	WORK	REST
Log Hop T-Stand	0:30	—
Diagonal Mountain Climber	0:30	—
Grasshopper	0:30	—
1-2 Push	0:30	—
REPEAT 3 ROUNDS		REST 30 SECONDS

SET 4

EXERCISE	WORK	REST
Pedal	0:30	—
Pelvic Peel	0:30	—
Pigeon Peel	0:30	—
Butterfly Peel	0:30	—
REPEAT 3 ROUNDS		REST 30 SECONDS

SET 5

EXERCISE	WORK	REST
Sphinx	0:30	—
Jumping Jack	0:30	—
Lizard Hop	0:30	—
Plus Jump	0:30	—
REPEAT 3 ROUNDS		REST 30 SECONDS

SET 6

EXERCISE	WORK	REST
Pike	0:30	—
Sprinter Sit-Up	0:30	—
Up and Overs	0:30	—
Plank	0:30	—
REPEAT 3 ROUNDS		REST 30 SECONDS

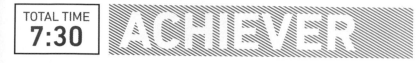

TOTAL TIME 7:30 — ACHIEVER

In order to reach your goals, you have to push beyond your comfort zone. This high-tempo, explosive routine will elevate you to the next level.

Do each exercise for 30 seconds. Rest 30 seconds after each round.

EXERCISE	WORK	REST
Squat Thrust	0:30	—
Burpee	0:30	—
Single Leg Burpee	0:30	—
Tuck Jump Burpee	0:30	—
REPEAT 3 ROUNDS		REST 30 SECONDS

TOTAL TIME 15:00 — FEEL THE BURN

This routine will have your legs screaming as the lactic acid builds and the burn increases. Stay strong and focused and you'll see results.

Do each exercise for 20 seconds. Rest 30 seconds after each round.

EXERCISE	WORK	REST
Squat	0:20	—
Reverse Lunge	0:20	—
Squat Jump	0:20	—
Pedal	0:20	—
Lateral Lunge	0:20	—
In and Outs	0:20	—
REPEAT 6 ROUNDS		REST 30 SECONDS

BY DESIGN

Build the body you've always wanted through hard work, dedication, and commitment. This head-to-toe HIIT routine will supply the foundation.

Do each exercise for 30 seconds. Do three rounds of each set. Rest 30 seconds after each round.

SET 1

EXERCISE	WORK	REST
Diagonal Mountain Climber	0:30	—
Tuck Jump	0:30	—
Pelvic Peel	0:30	—
V-Up	0:30	—
REPEAT 3 ROUNDS	REST 30 SECONDS	

SET 2

EXERCISE	WORK	REST
1-2 Push	0:30	—
Star	0:30	—
Squat Pedal	0:30	—
Flutter Up	0:30	—
REPEAT 3 ROUNDS	REST 30 SECONDS	

SET 3

EXERCISE	WORK	REST
Plyo Trio	0:30	—
Single Leg Burpee	0:30	—
Lateral Lift	0:30	—
Up and Overs	0:30	—
REPEAT 3 ROUNDS	REST 30 SECONDS	

DEDICATED

Dedication and commitment are the keys to your success. Put yourself to the test with this three-exercise set that will supercharge your metabolism.

Do each exercise for 20 seconds. Rest 30 seconds after each round.

EXERCISE	WORK	REST
Tuck Jump	0:20	—
Lizard Hop	0:20	—
Star	0:20	—
REPEAT 6 ROUNDS	REST 30 SECONDS	

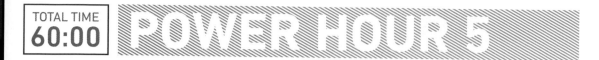

POWER HOUR 5

There are a lot of ways you can spend an hour, but few will be as challenging or rewarding as an hour of HIIT. Do 10 minutes of dynamic stretching before diving into the cardio warm-up.

WARM UP
5:00

WARM-UP

Before you push yourself to the max, get your body moving with a quick cardio warm-up.

EXERCISE	WORK	REST
Sprint	0:30	—
Jumping Jack	0:30	—
High Knees	0:30	—
X-Jack	0:30	—
Squat	0:30	—
REPEAT 2 ROUNDS		NO REST BETWEEN ROUNDS

WORKOUT
45:00

WORKOUT

This is the time to give it your all. It can be tough to maintain intensity for 45 minutes. Focus on form and build in more rest if you need to.

Do each exercise for 30 seconds. Do three rounds of each set. Rest 30 seconds after each round.

SET 1		
EXERCISE	WORK	REST
Plus Jump	0:30	—
Skater Jump	0:30	—
Log Hop T-Stand	0:30	—
1-2 Push	0:30	—
REPEAT 3 ROUNDS		REST 30 SECONDS

SET 2

EXERCISE	WORK	REST
Single Leg Peel (right)	0:30	—
Dragon Walk	0:30	—
Single Leg Peel (left)	0:30	—
Sprinter Sit-Up	0:30	—

REPEAT 3 ROUNDS — REST 30 SECONDS

SET 3

EXERCISE	WORK	REST
Squat Pedal	0:30	—
In and Outs	0:30	—
Tuck Jump Burpee	0:30	—
Reverse Push-Up	0:30	—

REPEAT 3 ROUNDS — REST 30 SECONDS

SET 4

EXERCISE	WORK	REST
Lizard Hop	0:30	—
Flutter-Up	0:30	—
Plyo Trio	0:30	—
Up and Overs	0:30	—

REPEAT 3 ROUNDS — REST 30 SECONDS

SET 5

EXERCISE	WORK	REST
Sphinx	0:30	—
Cross-Country Seal	0:30	—
Grasshopper	0:30	—
X-Jack	0:30	—

REPEAT 3 ROUNDS — REST 30 SECONDS

SET 6

EXERCISE	WORK	REST
Plank	0:30	—
Side Plank (right)	0:30	—
Plank	0:30	—
Side Plank (left)	0:30	—

REPEAT 3 ROUNDS — REST 30 SECONDS

No rest during this routine! Instead, this routine alternates high-impact exercises with lower-impact active recovery exercises, making sure that every second counts.

Do each exercise in order, alternating high-impact exercises with active recovery exercises. Go slowly during the active recovery exercises.

EXERCISE	WORK	ACTIVE RECOVERY	WORK
Sprint	0:30	Squat	0:30
Single Leg Burpee	0:30	Push-Up	0:30
Cross-Country Seal	0:30	Reverse Lunge	0:30
Tuck Jump	0:30	Peel	0:30
REPEAT 3 ROUNDS		NO REST BETWEEN ROUNDS	

HIIT can help you lose weight, increase your muscle tone, and gain strength, but it won't be easy. You have to be willing to work hard and build your body from the ground up, rep by rep, second by second.

Do each exercise for 30 seconds. Rest one minute after each round.

EXERCISE	WORK	REST
Plus Jump	0:30	—
Squat Pedal	0:30	—
Dragon Walk	0:30	—
Sprinter Sit-Up	0:30	—
Tuck Jump Burpee	0:30	—
Skater Jump	0:30	—
Reverse Push-Up	0:30	—
1-2 Push	0:30	—
REPEAT 3 ROUNDS		REST 1 MINUTE

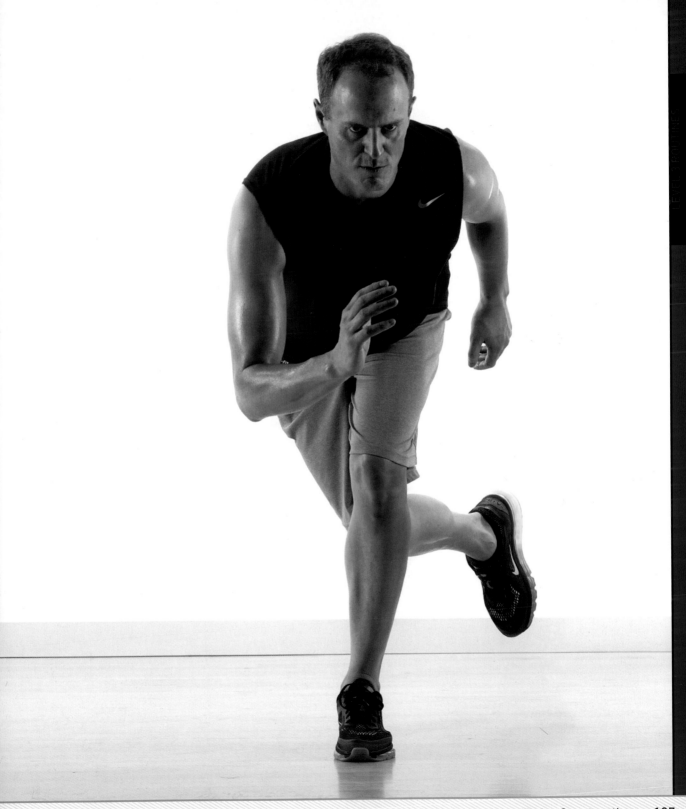

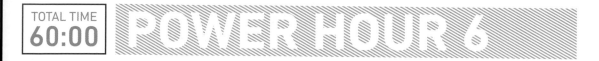

POWER HOUR 6

The last of the power-hour series of workouts includes six sets of some of the most popular HIIT exercises. Before you begin, do 10 minutes of dynamic stretching.

WARM UP
5:00

WARM-UP

Get your muscles warmed up with five minutes of cardio exercises. Work at 50 to 75 percent of your power.

EXERCISE	WORK	REST
Sprint	0:30	
Jumping Jack	0:30	
High Knees	0:30	
X-Jack	0:30	
Squat	0:30	
REPEAT 2 ROUNDS		NO REST BETWEEN ROUNDS

WORKOUT
45:00

WORKOUT

Push yourself for 45 minutes of high-intensity exercises. If you feel fatigued, increase the rest times between rounds.

Do each exercise for 30 seconds. Do three rounds of each set. Rest 30 seconds after each round.

SET 1		
EXERCISE	WORK	REST
Sprint	0:30	—
Squat Jump	0:30	—
Cross-Country Seal	0:30	—
1-2 Push	0:30	—
REPEAT 3 ROUNDS		REST 30 SECONDS

SET 2

EXERCISE	WORK	REST
Jumping Jack	0:30	—
Mountain Climber	0:30	—
Pedal	0:30	—
Spiderman	0:30	—
REPEAT 3 ROUNDS		REST 30 SECONDS

SET 3

EXERCISE	WORK	REST
Burpee	0:30	—
Squat Pedal	0:30	—
Triceps Dip	0:30	—
Reverse Push-Up	0:30	—
REPEAT 3 ROUNDS		REST 30 SECONDS

SET 4

EXERCISE	WORK	REST
High Knees	0:30	—
X-Jack	0:30	—
Lateral Lunge	0:30	—
Shoulder Press	0:30	—
REPEAT 3 ROUNDS		REST 30 SECONDS

SET 5

EXERCISE	WORK	REST
Sphinx	0:30	—
Plus Jump	0:30	—
Grasshopper	0:30	—
Tuck Jump	0:30	—
REPEAT 3 ROUNDS		REST 30 SECONDS

SET 6

EXERCISE	WORK	REST
Plank	0:30	—
Side Plank (right)	0:30	—
Sprinter Sit-Up	0:30	—
Side Plank (left)	0:30	—
REPEAT 3 ROUNDS		REST 30 SECONDS

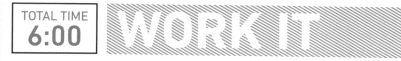

This simple, fun, and sweaty routine brings together three HIIT favorites, one from each level: sprints, squat jumps, and tuck jump burpees. Push for maximum heart rate, and remember: you get out what you put in.

Do each exercise for 30 seconds. Rest 30 seconds after each set.

EXERCISE	WORK	REST
Tuck Jump Burpee	0:30	—
Sprint	0:30	—
Squat Jump	0:30	—
↻ **REPEAT 3 ROUNDS**		REST 30 SECONDS

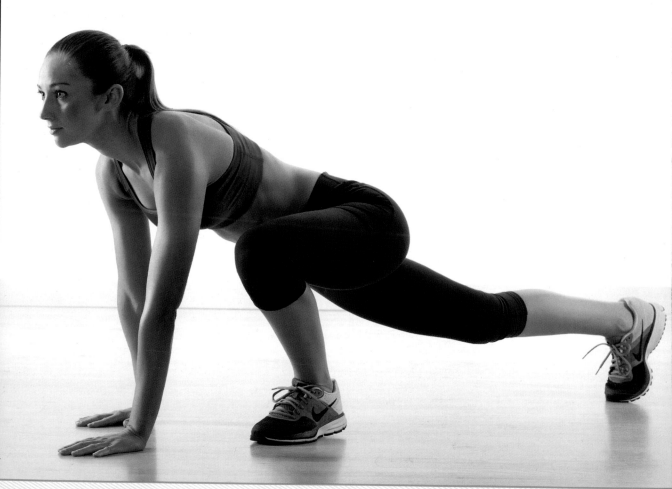

TOTAL TIME
12:00

GET RESULTS

In this routine, the work-to-rest ratio varies with each set. It will challenge your athleticism and strength, but the results and sense of achievement upon completion will be priceless.

Complete each set and rest for the specified time. Repeat the sequence three times.

SET 1		
EXERCISE	WORK	REST
High Knees	0:20	—
Jumping Jack	0:20	—
Tuck Jump	0:20	—
	REST 10 SECONDS	
SET 2		
Burpee	0:20	—
Lizard Hop	0:20	—
Star	0:20	—
	REST 20 SECONDS	
SET 3		
Sprint	0:20	—
Tuck Jump Burpee	0:20	—
1-2 Push	0:20	—
	REST 30 SECONDS	

🔁 **REPEAT 3 TIMES**

TOTAL TIME 9:00 — ONE STEP CLOSER

Each workout brings you one step closer to your goals. Stay committed and determined for this short, energetic routine that will challenge your entire body.

Do each exercise for 20 seconds. Rest 30 seconds after each round.

EXERCISE	WORK	REST
Plus Jump	0:20	—
Skater Jump	0:20	—
1-2 Push	0:20	—
REPEAT 6 ROUNDS		REST 30 SECONDS

TOTAL TIME 15:00 — GET FIT

HIIT gives you the tools to get fit, but it will take hard work and commitment to achieve your goals. Stay fast and focused for this explosive routine.

Do each exercise in order. Rest 30 seconds after each round.

EXERCISE	WORK	REST
Sprint	0:20	—
Tuck Jump	0:20	—
Diagonal Mountain Climber	0:20	—
Single Leg Burpee	0:20	—
Squat Pedal	0:20	—
Plyo Trio	0:20	—
REPEAT 6 ROUNDS		REST 30 SECONDS

The final Level 3 routine represents the HIIT philosophy: push hard and earn your sweat, enjoy your workouts with a smile, and repeat daily.

Do each round following the specified work-to-rest ratio. Rest one minute after each round.

TOTAL TIME
19:55

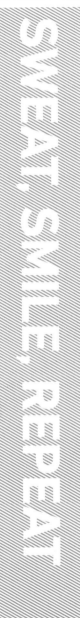

EXERCISE	ROUND 1		ROUND 2		ROUND 3	
	WORK	REST	WORK	REST	WORK	REST
Sprint	0:30	0:30	0:30	0:15	0:30	0:10
Squat Pedal	0:30	0:30	0:30	0:15	0:30	0:10
Diagonal Mountain Climber	0:30	0:30	0:30	0:15	0:30	0:10
Tuck Jump	0:30	0:30	0:30	0:15	0:30	0:10
Single Leg Burpee	0:30	0:30	0:30	0:15	0:30	0:10
1-2 Push	0:30	0:30	0:30	0:15	0:30	0:10
Plyo Push-Up	0:30	0:30	0:30	0:15	0:30	0:10
	REST 1 MINUTE		REST 1 MINUTE		REST 1 MINUTE	

3-DAY CHALLENGE

This short but intense introduction to HIIT is the perfect way to shake up your weekly workout routine or kick off a weight-loss program. Commit to three days of HIIT and you'll start to feel a difference!

DAY	ROUTINE
1	Sweat, Smile, Repeat
2	Power Hour 1
3	Power Hour 2

TRAINER TIPS

- Before starting your HIIT routine, do a few minutes of dynamic stretching as a warm-up.

- Review the exercises in each routine and make sure you know how to do them properly before beginning a workout.

- In addition to your workout challenge, challenge yourself to make healthy eating choices. Monitoring your caloric intake will help you make the most of HIIT.

This week-long challenge features a blend of short and long sets, plyometrics, compound strength exercises, and core-building exercises to kick your workouts into high gear. After just one week of HIIT, you'll begin to feel stronger and more energized.

DAY	ROUTINE
1	Work It
2	Power Hour 2
3	Redline
4	Power Hour 4
5	Drop Sets
6	Power Hour 6
7	Killer Cardio

TRAINER TIPS

- Warm up before each routine with three to five minutes of dynamic stretching.
- Choosing a consistent time and place to do your HIIT workouts will make it easier to make them part of your daily routine.
- If you experience soreness the day after working out, use a foam roller to facilitate myofascial release.

After two weeks of HIIT, you should see results! The routines in this program will help you lose weight, build strength, and improve cardiovascular endurance with a combination of body weight and plyometric exercises. The first week will get you acclimated to HIIT, and the second week takes it up a notch with longer and more challenging routines.

DAY	ROUTINE
1	Hard Charger
2	Full Throttle
3	Level Up
4	High Five
5	Heavy HIIT-er
6	Conquer
7	Posture Perfect

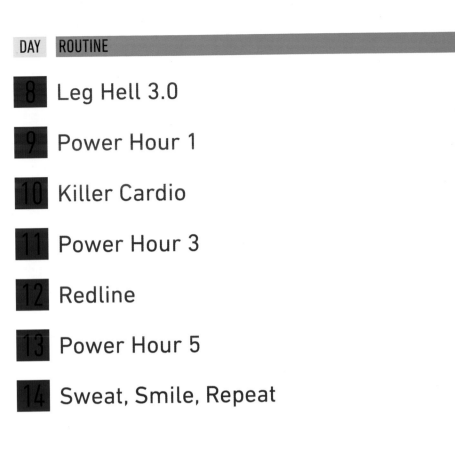

DAY	ROUTINE
8	Leg Hell 3.0
9	Power Hour 1
10	Killer Cardio
11	Power Hour 3
12	Redline
13	Power Hour 5
14	Sweat, Smile, Repeat

 TRAINER TIPS

- Remember that quality is more important than quantity. The 14-Day Challenge introduces more athletic exercises, which means attention to form is critical.

- Stay mentally strong and focus on your goals. Two weeks takes dedication. It's easy for "just one day off" to turn into two and then three. Stick with it.

- Be aware of what you eat. You'll see greater changes if you are disciplined in your eating as well as your exercise.

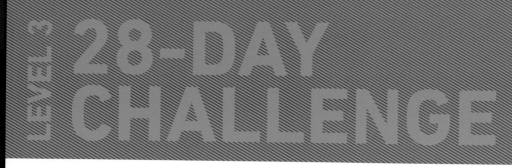

28-DAY CHALLENGE

This four-week workout plan features a variety of routine styles and formats to keep things interesting, fun, and intense. The length and difficulty of the routines increases each week, ensuring that you're always challenged. Monitor your progress by completing the fitness assessment every two weeks.

DAY	ROUTINE
1	Achiever
2	Feel the Burn
3	Every Second Counts
4	Defined
5	Hard Charger
6	Conquer
7	Level Up

DAY	ROUTINE
8	Full Throttle
9	Posture Perfect
10	Get Results
11	Under Construction
12	One Step Closer
13	Get Fit
14	Drop Sets

DAY	ROUTINE
15	Sweat and Smile
16	Heavy HIIT-er
17	Be Agile
18	Killer Cardio
19	High Five
20	Challenge = Change
21	Redline

DAY	ROUTINE
22	Power Hour 1
23	Power Hour 2
24	Power Hour 3
25	Power Hour 4
26	Power Hour 5
27	Power Hour 6
28	Smile, Sweat, Repeat

TRAINER TIPS

- For top performance and injury prevention, warm up with dynamic stretching before beginning your workout.

- If you've been using a regular timer to measure the time increments for your workouts, try switching to an app that allows you to program specific intervals, such as Interval Timer Pro.

- Recovery is important, especially when you're working out daily. Stay hydrated during your workouts, and use a foam roller to alleviate muscle pain.

- If you're making the commitment to do HIIT for 28 days, commit to monitoring your diet as well. Getting the results you want takes discipline.

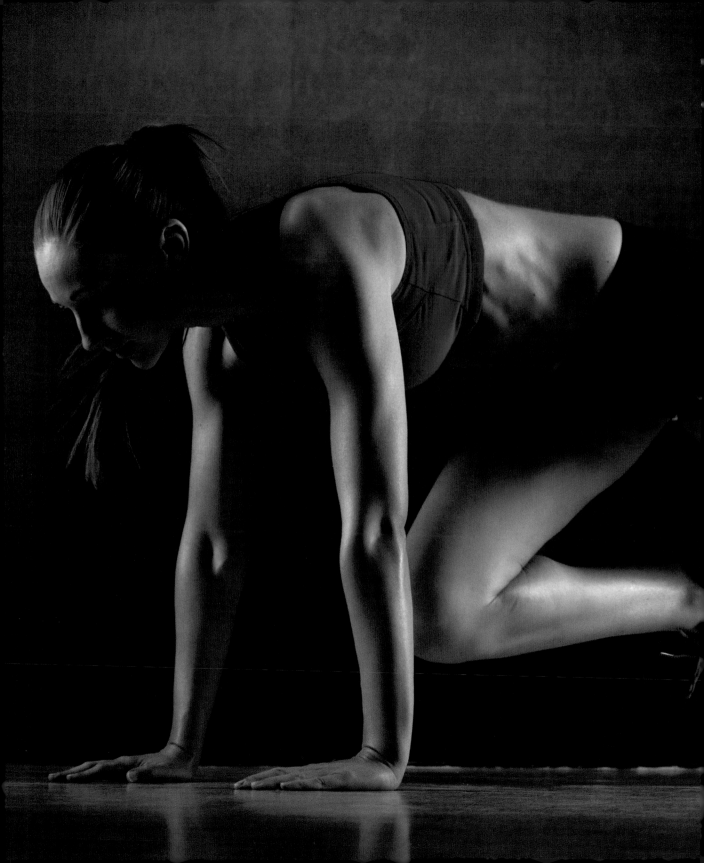

Cardio exercise is defined as any exercise that increases the work of the heart and lungs, raising your heart rate. The exercises in this part will get you sweating with a variety of formats including short, incendiary exercises, such as the sprint; multiplanar exercises, such as the cross-country seal; and explosive plyometric exercises, such as the burpee. Check the leveled progression guide for each exercise. If a movement is too simple, try the next level up. If you're struggling, try the next level down.

SQUAT THRUST

The difference between a burpee and squat thrust is a topic of some debate, but in my studio, a burpee includes a push-up and a jump while the squat thrust does not. That doesn't mean it's easier, though. Fewer steps means you can do more reps!

PROGRESSION

LEVEL 1:	**Squat Thrust**
LEVEL 2:	Burpee
LEVEL 3:	Single Leg Burpee

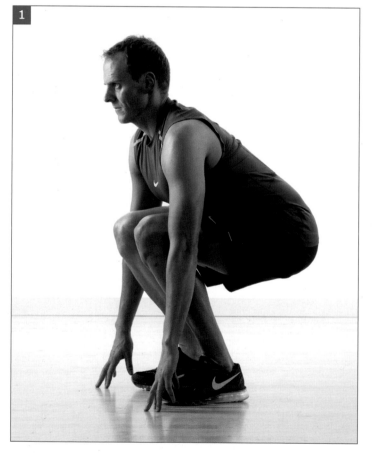

With your feet hip width apart, bend your knees and bring your hands to the floor just in front of your feet.

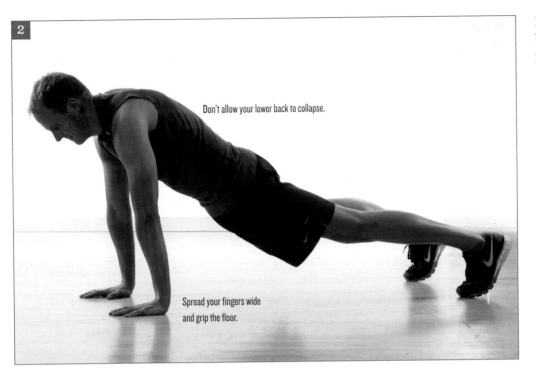

2

Don't allow your lower back to collapse.

Spread your fingers wide and grip the floor.

Hop your feet back into a plank position.

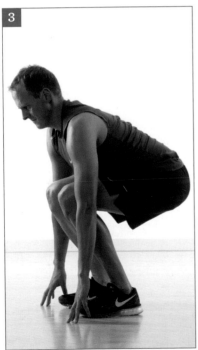

3

Jump your feet back to your hands, shifting your weight into the heels and lifting your chest.

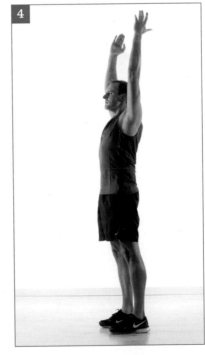

4

Stand up, tucking the pelvis, engaging the abs, and extending the arms above your head. Repeat as quickly as possible while maintaining proper form.

HIGH KNEES

This is an excellent exercise for runners and athletes who wish to improve running form and foot speed. The dynamic running motion will challenge your cardiovascular endurance and help to strengthen your hip flexors.

PROGRESSION

LEVEL 1:	**High Knees**
LEVEL 2:	Tuck Jump
LEVEL 3:	Tuck Jump Burpee

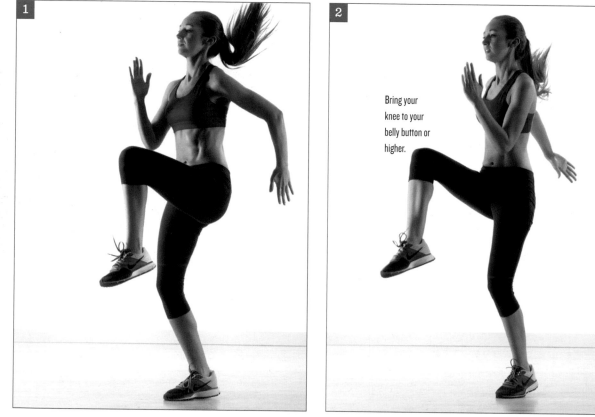

Bring your knee to your belly button or higher.

Stand with feet hip width apart. Drive your right knee toward your chest and quickly place it back on the ground.

Immediately follow by driving the left knee to the chest. Alternate knees as quickly as you can. The movement is similar to jogging in place, but you bring your knees higher. Keep your chest up, shoulders back, and core engaged.

MOUNTAIN CLIMBER

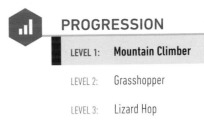

PROGRESSION

LEVEL 1:	**Mountain Climber**
LEVEL 2:	Grasshopper
LEVEL 3:	Lizard Hop

Mountain climbers strengthen your core, hip flexors, and legs and provide an intense cardio challenge. Drive your knees toward your chest as quickly as possible to maximize the cardiovascular benefits.

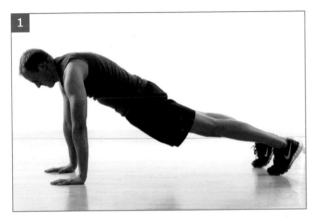

Position your hands on the floor slightly wider than shoulder width apart. Rise up onto your toes and engage the core to form a straight line between your ankles and head.

CHALLENGE

Try elevating your hands on a small step, bench, or a stability ball to increase the difficulty level of this exercise.

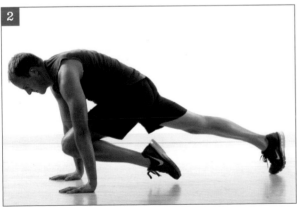

Bring your left knee in toward your chest, engaging your core. Attempt to pull your knee all the way through your supporting arms to maximize engagement of the core.

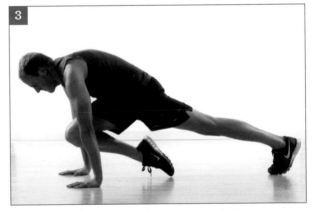

Quickly extend the left leg and simultaneously pull the right knee toward the chest. Repeat with controlled speed.

SPRINT

Sprinting is a simple and effective means of elevating your heart rate and burning fat. This high-intensity exercise can be done in place or back and forth across an open space. Keep moving quickly to maximize the cardio benefits.

PROGRESSION

LEVEL 1: **Sprint**

LEVEL 2: Cross-Country Seal

LEVEL 3: Plus Jump

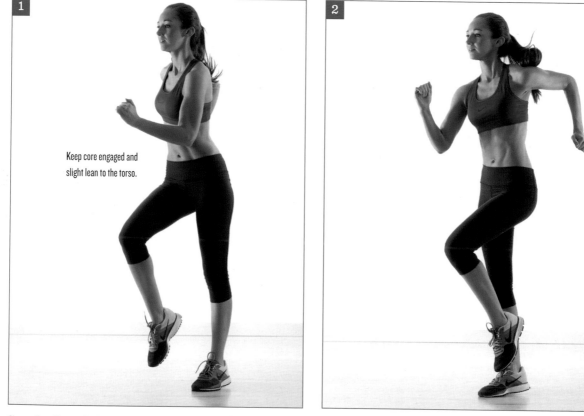

Keep core engaged and slight lean to the torso.

Stand tall, with feet shoulder width apart and a slight lean to the body. Drive your right knee to your chest as your left arm swings forward.

As your right leg lowers, drive forward with your left knee and right arm. Repeat with control, always moving opposite arms and legs.

JUMPING JACK

Jumping jacks are one of the most familiar and effective cardio exercises out there. This explosive move is a great way to improve cardiovascular endurance and also engage the core, shoulders, back, and calves.

PROGRESSION

LEVEL 1:	**Jumping Jack**
LEVEL 2:	X-Jack
LEVEL 3:	Star

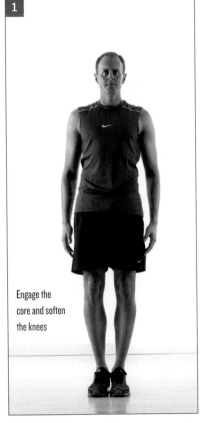

1

Engage the core and soften the knees

Stand with your feet together and your arms at your sides.

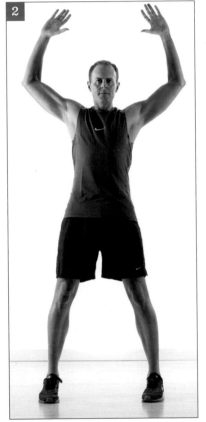

2

Jump up as you spread your feet wide and raise your arms overhead in a V-shape. Land with your feet spread and arms up.

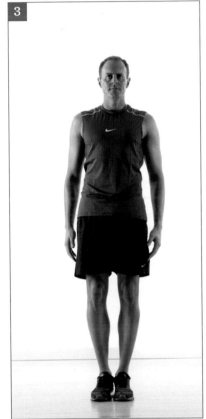

3

Jump again, bringing your feet together and returning your arms to the sides. Repeat.

BURPEE

The burpee is indisputably the ultimate total-body exercise. Each one will work your chest, arms, shoulders, thighs, hamstrings, and core. Burpees can be intimidating, but the benefits are worth the challenge.

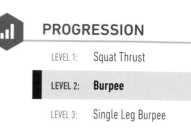

PROGRESSION

LEVEL 1:   Squat Thrust

LEVEL 2:   **Burpee**

LEVEL 3:   Single Leg Burpee

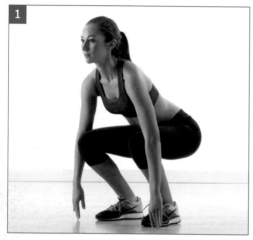

With your feet hip width apart, bend your knees and bring your hands to the floor just in front of your feet.

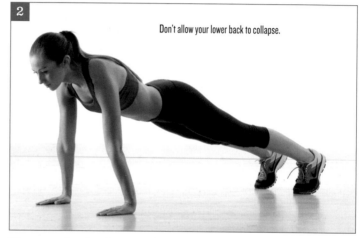

Don't allow your lower back to collapse.

Hop your feet back into a plank position. Spread your fingers wide and grip the floor.

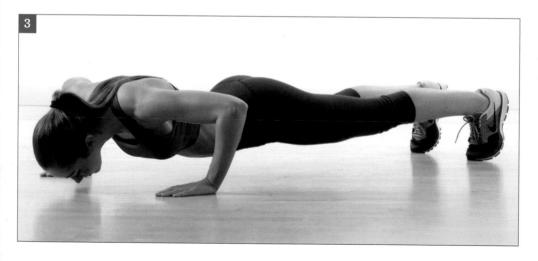

Perform one push-up with your core engaged.

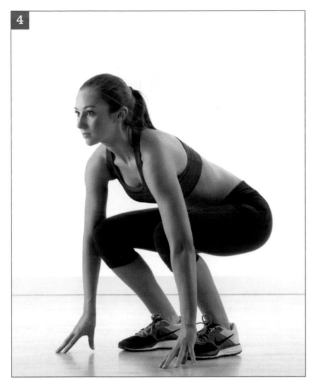

4

Jump your feet back to your hands, shifting your weight into the heels and lifting your chest.

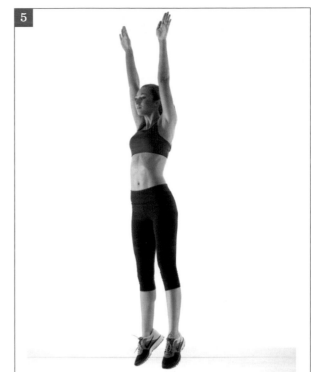

5

Jump up from the crouched position and reach overhead with your hands.

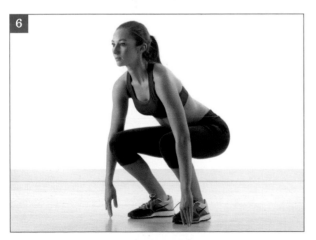

6

Land softly with a slight bend at your knees, hips, and ankles. Repeat.

CHALLENGE

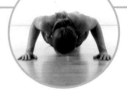

Substitute the regular push-up with a triceps push-up, keeping your elbows tight to your rib cage.

TUCK JUMP

Tuck jumps are an intense, plyometric move that will drive your heart rate through the roof while working the muscles in your core and legs. The explosive nature of the exercise will improve agility and power.

PROGRESSION

LEVEL 1:   High Knees

LEVEL 2:   **Tuck Jump**

LEVEL 3:   Tuck Jump Burpee

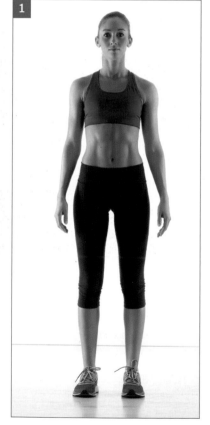

1

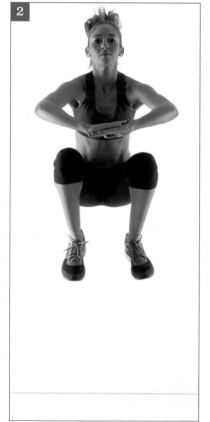

2

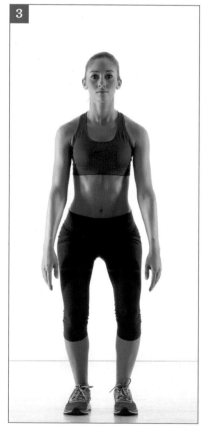

3

Stand tall with your knees slightly bent.

Quickly lower into a half squat and immediately explode upward. Jump as high as you can, driving your knees toward the chest and attempting to touch them to the palms of your hands.

Land softly, absorbing the impact by bending at the ankles, knees, and hips to decelerate the body.

GRASSHOPPER

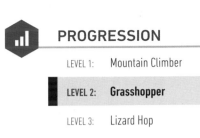

PROGRESSION

LEVEL 1:   Mountain Climber

LEVEL 2:   **Grasshopper**

LEVEL 3:   Lizard Hop

The grasshopper's powerful legs are the inspiration for this exercise. This move will torch the thighs, core, and shoulders while increasing athletic performance and hip mobility. Move as quickly as you can while maintaining proper form.

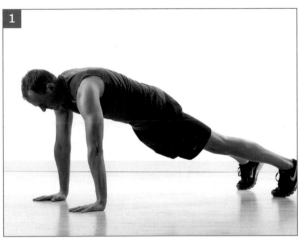

Assume a plank position. Your elbows should be directly beneath your shoulders and your body should form a straight line from head to heels.

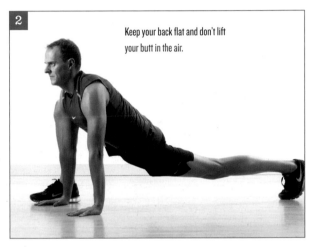

Keep your back flat and don't lift your butt in the air.

Bring your right foot forward, and place it on the floor just outside of your right hand.

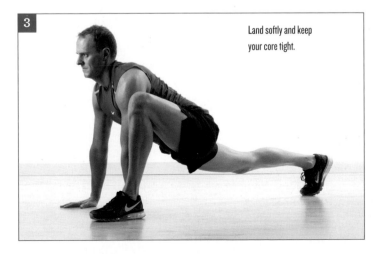

Land softly and keep your core tight.

Jump and switch the feet, landing with the left foot on the floor just outside of the left hand. Repeat, alternating legs with controlled speed.

CROSS-COUNTRY SEAL

■ PROGRESSION

LEVEL 1: Sprint

LEVEL 2: **Cross-Country Seal**

LEVEL 3: Plus Jump

This exercise mimics the motion of cross-country skiing, and improves cardiovascular endurance by working all the major muscle groups of the body. The cross-country seal opens the arms laterally, creating a multi-planar exercise that targets the shoulders, back, legs, and glutes.

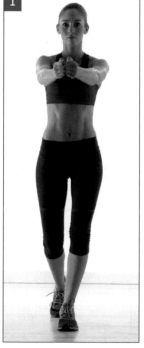

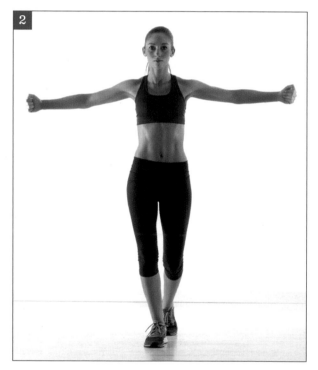

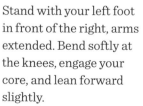

1 Stand with your left foot in front of the right, arms extended. Bend softly at the knees, engage your core, and lean forward slightly.

2 Jump and switch feet, opening your arms and squeezing your shoulder blades while in the air. Land softly, with your right foot in front of the left.

3 Jump and switch feet again, returning to the starting position with your arms in front of you. Repeat with controlled speed.

X-JACK

This innovative twist on the traditional jumping jack will boost your metabolism and tone your legs, core, shoulders, and back.

PROGRESSION

LEVEL 1:   Jumping Jack

LEVEL 2:   **X-Jack**

LEVEL 3:   Star

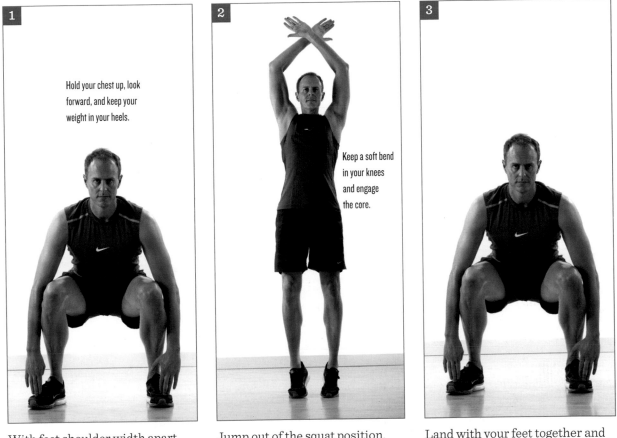

1 Hold your chest up, look forward, and keep your weight in your heels.

2 Keep a soft bend in your knees and engage the core.

3

With feet shoulder width apart, bend from your hips, knees, and ankles and drop into a squat position. If you can, touch your toes with your fingertips

Jump out of the squat position. As you jump, extend your legs and raise your arms overhead, crossing your wrists to make an X.

Land with your feet together and your weight on the balls of your feet. Lower back to the squat position and repeat.

SINGLE LEG BURPEE

PROGRESSION

LEVEL 1:   Squat Thrust

LEVEL 2:   Burpee

LEVEL 3:   **Single Leg Burpee**

In this modification of the traditional burpee, you raise one leg throughout the plank and push-up phase of the exercise. The increased load challenges your abdominals, lower back, and stabilizing leg.

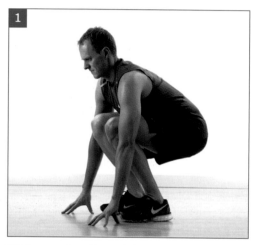

With your feet hip width apart, bend your knees and bring your hands to the floor just in front of your feet.

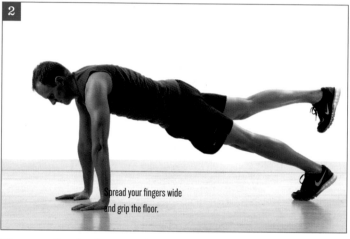

Spread your fingers wide and grip the floor.

Hop your feet back into a plank position with one leg lifted off the floor to shoulder height.

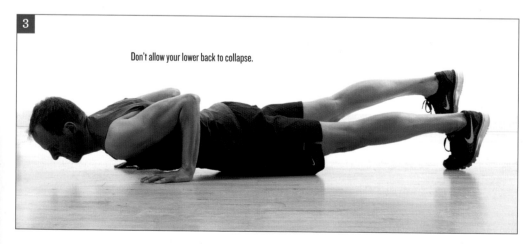

Don't allow your lower back to collapse.

Perform one push-up with your core engaged and leg elevated.

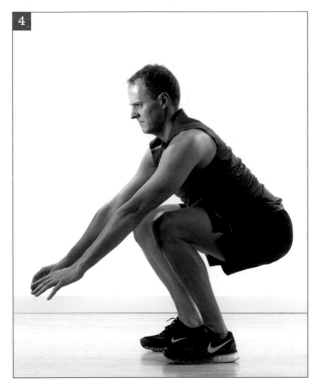

Lower the leg and jump your feet back to your hands, shifting your weight into the heels and lifting your chest.

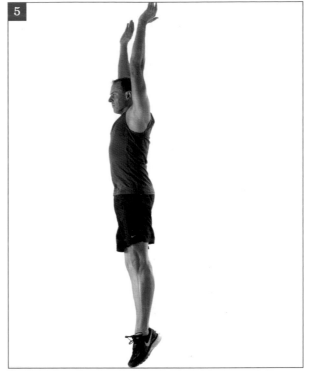

Jump up from the crouched position and reach overhead with your hands.

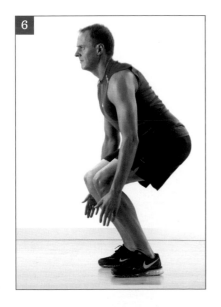

Land softly with a slight bend at your knees, hips, and ankles. Repeat, alternating the elevated leg with each rep.

 CHALLENGE

For added challenge, substitute the regular push-up with a triceps push-up, keeping your elbows tight to your rib cage.

TUCK JUMP BURPEE

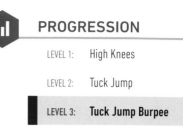

PROGRESSION

LEVEL 1: High Knees

LEVEL 2: Tuck Jump

LEVEL 3: **Tuck Jump Burpee**

The tuck jump and the burpee, two of the toughest exercises in this book, combine to create an incredible cardiovascular and strength exercise reserved only for those feeling superhuman.

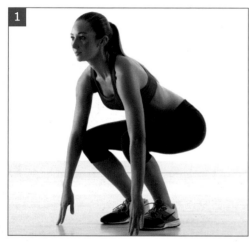

With your feet hip width apart, bend your knees and bring hands to the floor just in front of your feet.

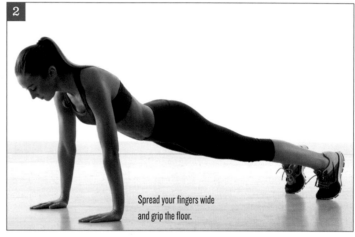

Spread your fingers wide and grip the floor.

Hop your feet back into a plank position

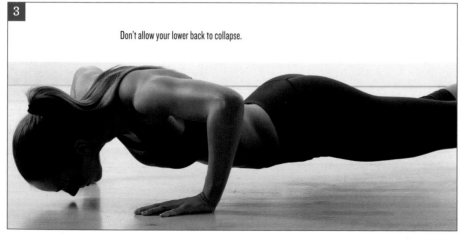

Don't allow your lower back to collapse.

Perform one push-up with your core engaged.

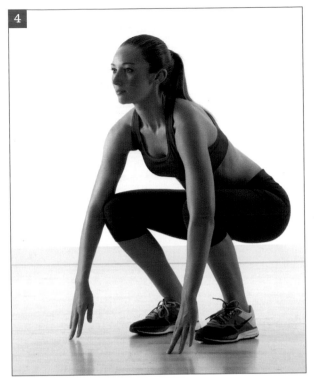

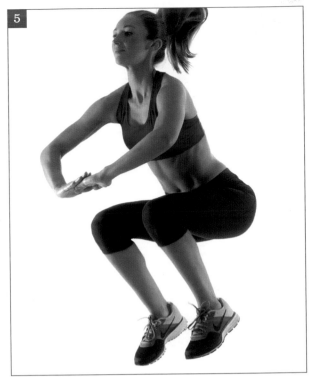

Jump your feet back to your hands, shifting your weight into the heels and lifting your chest.

Jump up from the crouched position and tuck your knees to your chest.

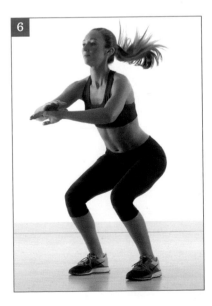

Land softly with a slight bend at your knees, hips, and ankles. Repeat.

 CHALLENGE

For added challenge, substitute the regular push-up with a triceps push-up, keeping your elbows tight to your rib cage.

LIZARD HOP

This explosive exercise builds upper-body strength, increases hip mobility, and creates core stability. Keep your movements quick and controlled to gain the most benefit.

PROGRESSION

LEVEL 1:   Mountain Climber

LEVEL 2:   Grasshopper

LEVEL 3:   **Lizard Hop**

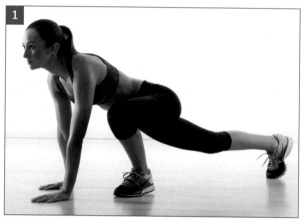

Begin in a staggered push-up position with your left hand ahead of right. Bend your left leg so that your foot is on the floor slightly to the side of the left hip.

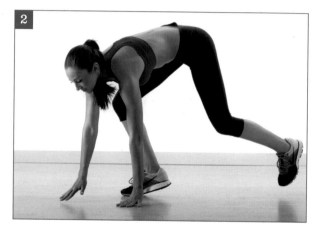

Bend your elbows slightly and engage your core. Imagine loading a spring full of energy and then explode, pressing through the floor and switching your hands and feet in the air.

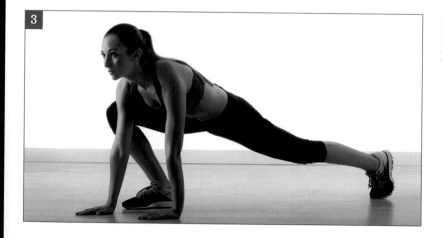

Land softly with your right hand in front of the left, and your right leg bent.

STAR

This plyometric powerhouse combines the squat jump and the jumping jack, resulting in a challenging exercise that will get your heart pumping and your quads burning.

PROGRESSION

LEVEL 1: Jumping Jack

LEVEL 2: X-Jack

LEVEL 3: **Star**

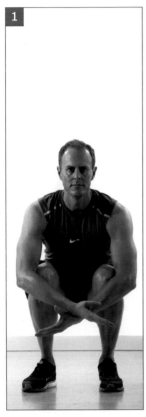

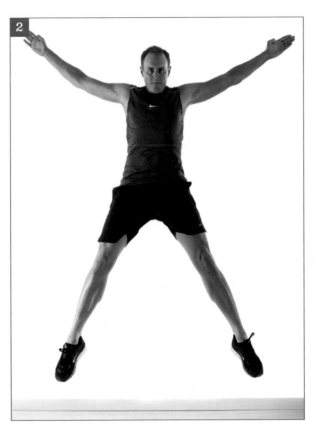

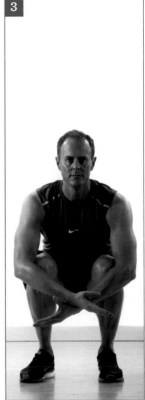

With your body weight in your heels, inhale as you bend at the knee, lowering into a squat position and wrapping your arms loosely around your shins.

Engage your core and exhale as you jump and explode through your heels into the air. Open your arms and legs as wide as you can, making a "star" shape.

Land as softly and silently as possible, bending slightly at the hips, knees, and ankles to decelerate the body.

PLUS JUMP

Small, plyometric hops from front to back and from side to side elevate the heart rate, super-charge the metabolism, and strengthen the ankles. This is a great exercise for building agility and foot speed.

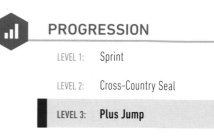

PROGRESSION

LEVEL 1:   Sprint

LEVEL 2:   Cross-Country Seal

LEVEL 3:   **Plus Jump**

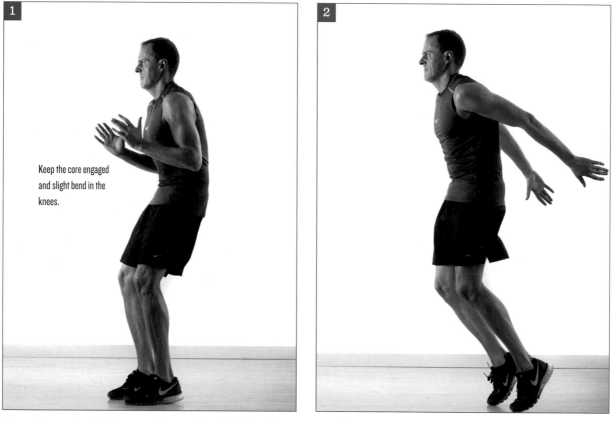

1 Keep the core engaged and slight bend in the knees.

Jump forward with feet together and a slight bend in the knees.

2

Quickly jump backward, landing softly with the core engaged. Jump forward and back a total of four times.

Try hopping on one leg at a time, switching legs after you've repeated the sequence four times.

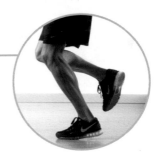

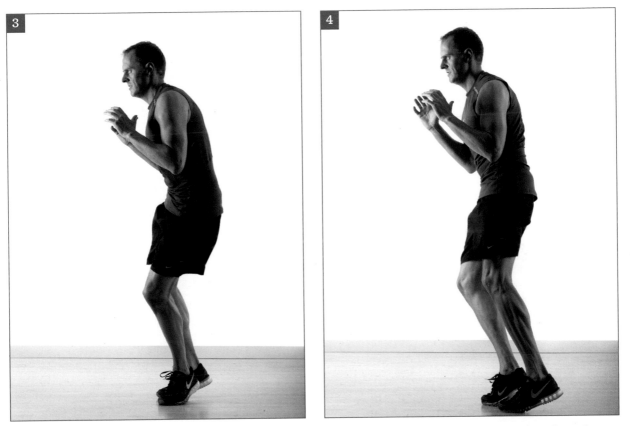

Jump to the right, keeping the soft bend in the knees and core engaged for balance.

Quickly jump to the left and then back to the right. Jump side to side a total of four times. Move as fast as possible to keep your heart rate up.

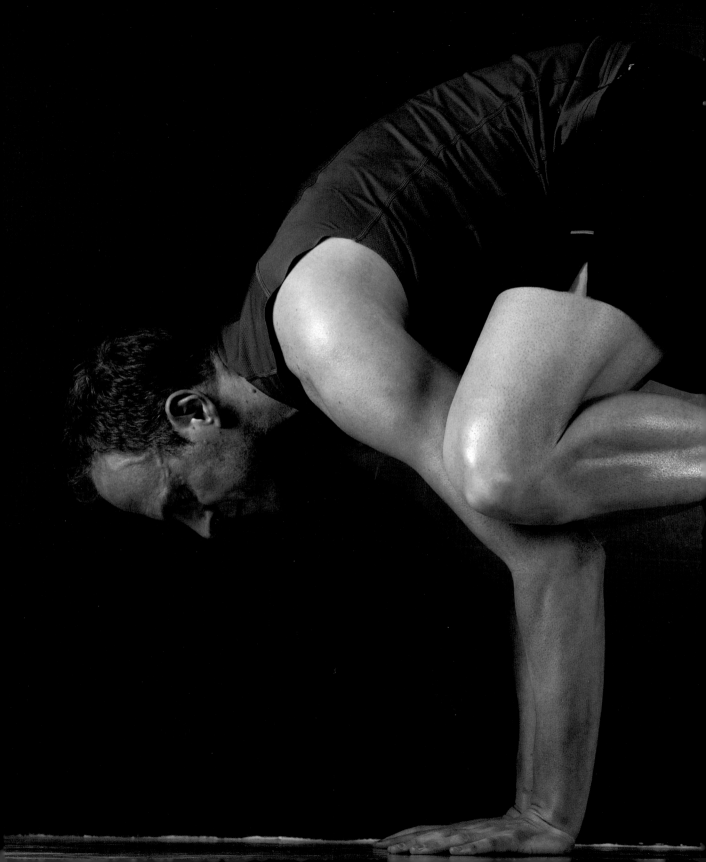

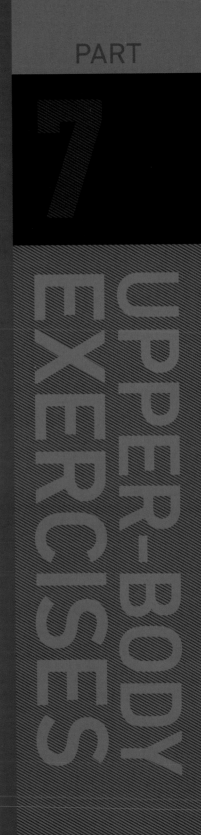

PART

7

UPPER-BODY EXERCISES

The exercises in this part focus on the muscles of the upper body, including the shoulders, back, chest, triceps, and core. They are designed to increase muscle tone and definition while building strength and stability. Check the leveled progression guide for each exercise and modify your routine as needed by selecting a similar exercise that is more or less difficult based on your needs.

KNEELING PUSH-UP

This modified push-up builds upper-body and core strength using the muscles of the chest, back, shoulders, triceps, abs, and even the legs. It's a great way to develop the strength required to tackle a full push-up, as well as an excellent substitute for those with compromised wrists or shoulders.

PROGRESSION

LEVEL 1:	**Kneeling Push-Up**
LEVEL 2:	Push-Up
LEVEL 3:	Plyo Push-Up

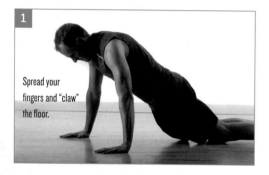

Spread your fingers and "claw" the floor.

Begin on all fours with your shoulders directly over your wrists. Tilt your pelvis and lower your hips until your body forms a straight line from knees to shoulders.

TRAINER TIP

To speed your progression to regular push-ups, hold the pause at the deepest part of your push-up. This will help develop strength in your shoulders, chest, and back.

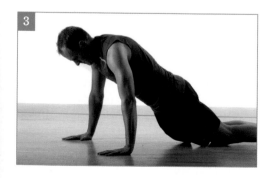

Bend your elbows, bringing your chest toward the floor. When your elbows are bent slightly beyond 90 degrees, hold for one to two seconds.

TRAINER TIP

Both kneeling and traditional push-ups engage the rotator cuff, posterior deltoids, rhomboids, abs, and the serratus anterior. Traditional push-ups with straight legs work more muscles in your lower body, involving your glutes and quadriceps as stabilizers throughout the movement. If you modify traditional push-ups by kneeling, add squats or T-stands to your workout to target the lower body.

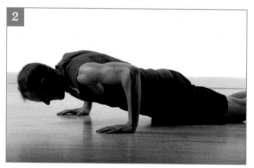

Push up through your palms, extending the arms to return to the starting position.

TRICEPS DIP

This targeted exercise is specifically designed to strengthen and define your triceps. The triceps run along the humerus (the main bone in your upper arm) between the shoulder and elbow. Along with the biceps, they aid in extension and retraction of the forearm and in the stabilization of the shoulder joint.

PROGRESSION

LEVEL 1:	**Triceps Dip**
LEVEL 2:	Military Push-Up
LEVEL 3:	Sphinx

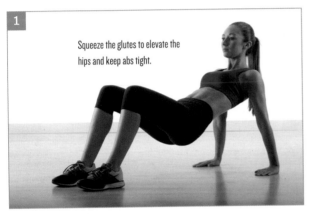

1

Squeeze the glutes to elevate the hips and keep abs tight.

Sit with your feet flat on the floor in front of you and knees slightly bent. Lean back slightly and place your hands on the floor behind your hips, fingers pointing toward your toes. Elevate the hips by engaging the core, hamstrings, and glutes.

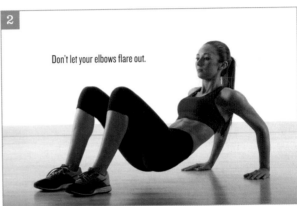

2

Don't let your elbows flare out.

Bend your elbows, lowering your hips until they're just above the floor.

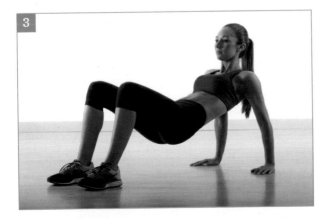

3

Extend your arms, bringing your hips back up to the starting position. Repeat.

TRAINER TIP

For a deeper movement, you can do triceps dips with your hands on a stable, elevated surface, such as a bench.

SHOULDER PRESS JACK

This twist on the classic jumping jack focuses on the *latissimus dorsi,* or lats, the largest muscles in your back. Concentrate on keeping the lats engaged and use explosive movements to boost your heart rate.

PROGRESSION

LEVEL 1: **Shoulder Press Jack**

LEVEL 2: Shoulder Press

LEVEL 3: Reverse Push-Up

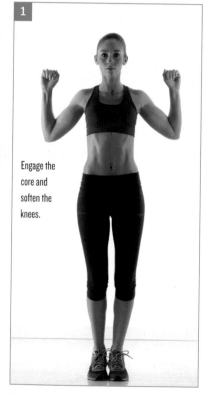

Engage the core and soften the knees.

Stand with your feet together and your hands up, with elbows by your sides. Make your hands into fists and concentrate on engaging your lats.

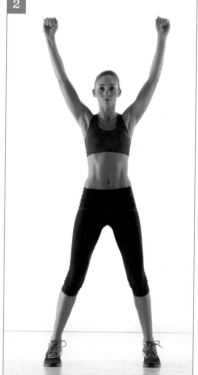

Jump up, opening your feet wider than your shoulders and simultaneously punching your arms toward the roof.

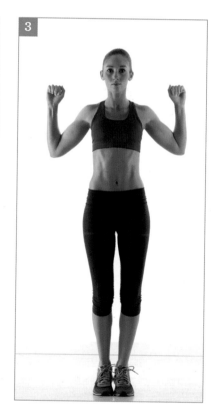

Jump again, bringing the feet together as you tuck your elbows into your sides and concentrate on squeezing and engaging the lats. Repeat.

SIDE PRESS

The side press isolates the shoulders and triceps, making it an excellent way to build upper-body strength.

PROGRESSION

LEVEL 1:	**Side Press**
LEVEL 2:	Side Plank Push-Up
LEVEL 3:	Plyo Trio

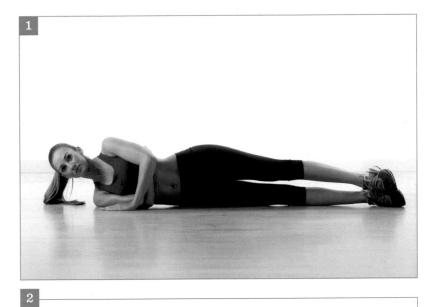

1

Lie on your side with your bottom arm wrapped around your core. Your top arm should be placed with your hand flat on the floor and your elbow at a 90-degree angle in front of your chest.

2

Press body as high off the floor as possible and engage the obliques.

Push through your top hand to lift your shoulders and torso off the ground, and then lower back down. Repeat.

CHALLENGE

For an added challenge, lift the top leg as you press. Elevating the leg will work your glutes, abductors, adductors, and obliques.

INCHWORM

This full-body exercise works the arms, chest, back, and core. As your body inches along the floor, it mimics the up-and-down motion of a moving inchworm.

PROGRESSION

LEVEL 1: **Inchworm**

LEVEL 2: Spiderman

LEVEL 3: Dragon Walk

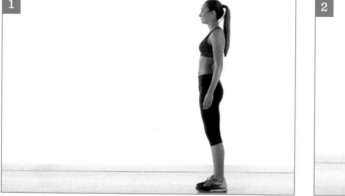

Stand tall with straight legs.

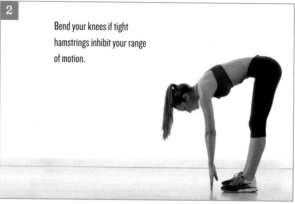

Bend your knees if tight hamstrings inhibit your range of motion.

Fold forward from the hips and bend over to touch the floor.

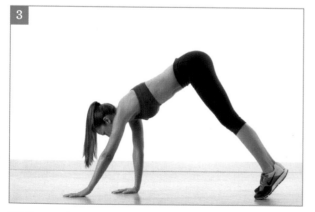

Walk your hands forward one at a time.

TRAINER TIP

If you have limited space, do the inchworm in place. Walk your hands forward, then reverse the movement and walk your hands backward.

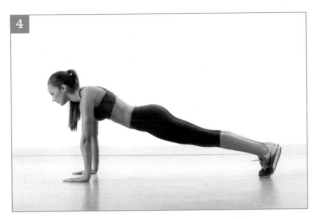

Stop when you reach a plank position, with your hands under your shoulders.

CHALLENGE

For an even greater challenge to your arms and shoulders, do a push-up or diagonal mountain climbers after you walk out your arms.

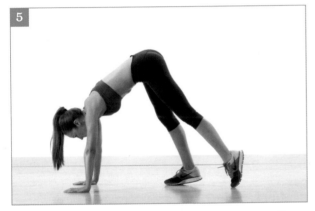

Walk your feet forward one at a time, taking small steps.

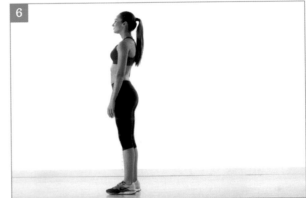

When your feet meet your hands, engage your core and roll up your spine to finish in the starting position.

CHALLENGE

Add a weight plate. Place a weight plate under your toes, forcing you to pull the weight simultaneously with both the feet to the hands. This increases the work load for the quads and core.

Add a gliding disk. Use a gliding disk (or paper plate on carpeted floors) to make the exercise more cardiovascular and fluid, elevating the heart rate and burning a few more calories.

PUSH-UP

The push-up may be the perfect compound exercise. If done correctly, it builds upper-body and core strength using the muscles of the chest, back, shoulders, triceps, abs, and even the legs. Keep an eye on your form.

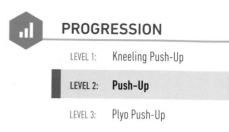

PROGRESSION

LEVEL 1:	Kneeling Push-Up
LEVEL 2:	**Push-Up**
LEVEL 3:	Plyo Push-Up

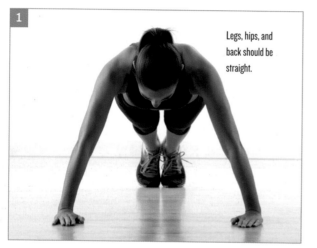

Legs, hips, and back should be straight.

Begin on all fours and position your hands on the floor slightly wider than shoulder width apart. Extend your legs and rise up onto your toes, engaging your core and forming a straight line from ankles to head.

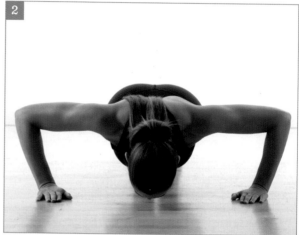

Bend your elbows, bringing your chest toward the floor. Once your elbows are bent slightly beyond 90 degrees, push up through your hands, extending the arms to return to the starting position.

 CHALLENGE

There are many push-up variations to try. Try adjusting the position of your hands to work slightly different muscle groups and make the move more challenging.

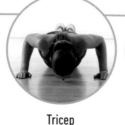

Tricep

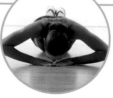

Heart to Hands

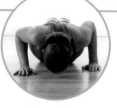

Staggered

MILITARY PUSH-UP

PROGRESSION

LEVEL 1: Triceps Dip

LEVEL 2: **Military Push-Up**

LEVEL 3: Sphinx

The military push-up changes the hand positioning of the traditional push-up, which puts more pressure on the triceps. It's a great way to strengthen and tone your arms, as well as your core and shoulders.

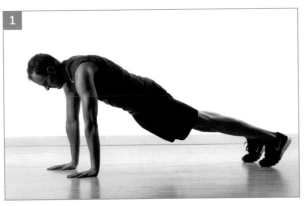

Assume a traditional push-up position with your core engaged and your body in a straight line between the head and ankles. Position your hands directly under your shoulders. Your hands should not be wider than the shoulders.

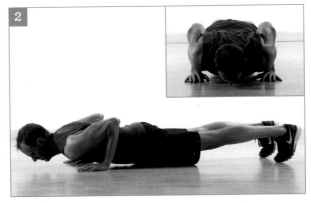

Lower your chest toward the floor, keeping your elbows and arms tight to your sides.

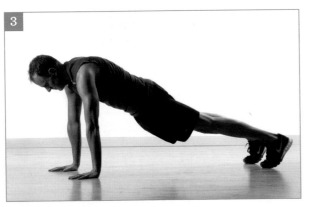

Push up through your hands, extending the arms to return to the starting position.

 CAUTION

Due to the increased load on the triceps, military push-ups are difficult to perform with correct form. If you feel your hips lifting while doing the exercise, switch to a traditional push-up or perform the military push-ups on your knees.

PIKE PUSH-UP

Pike push-ups are one of the best body weight exercises you can do to build shoulder strength and also the precursor to handstand push-ups.

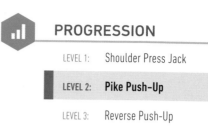

PROGRESSION

LEVEL 1:	Shoulder Press Jack
LEVEL 2:	**Pike Push-Up**
LEVEL 3:	Reverse Push-Up

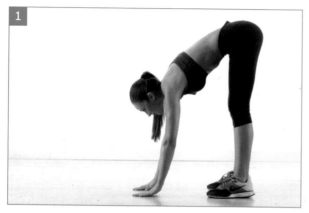

Stand tall and then fold forward from the hips until your hands are on the floor.

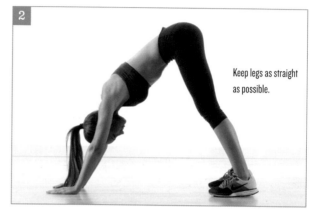

Keep legs as straight as possible.

Walk hands away from the body until you form a triangle with the ground. The further your hands are from the feet, the easier the exercise becomes, as you can use the muscles of the chest and back to assist the shoulders.

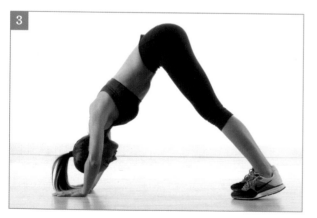

Bend your arms and lower the crown of your head to the floor. Your arms should form approximately a 90-degree angle. Extend the arms and repeat.

TRAINER TIP

This exercise becomes more difficult as you move your feet closer to your hands, because you are pressing a greater proportion of body weight. Adjust how close your feet are to your hands to vary the difficulty level.

SPIDERMAN

This variation on the push-up is inspired by the agile superhero of the same name. It will increase hip mobility and flexibility and build core strength.

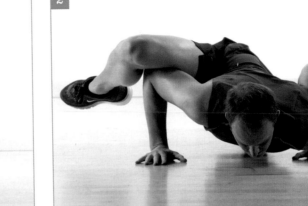

Assume a standard push-up position, with palms just wider than shoulders, arms straight, and body in a straight line balanced between arms and toes.

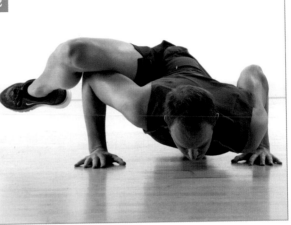

Bend your arms, bringing the chest down as you lift your right foot off the floor. Swing the right leg out sideways, bringing your right knee up toward your right shoulder.

Bring your right foot back to the floor and push your body back to the starting position. Repeat, alternating legs.

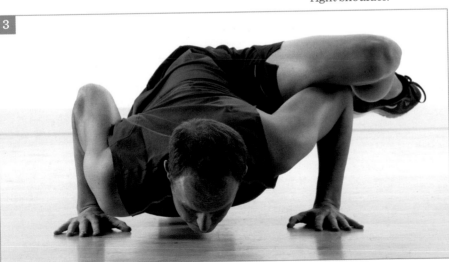

SIDE PLANK PUSH-UP

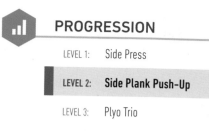

PROGRESSION

LEVEL 1:   Side Press

LEVEL 2:   **Side Plank Push-Up**

LEVEL 3:   Plyo Trio

The side plank push-up is an excellent way to isolate the shoulders and triceps while engaging the obliques for stabilization. Correct hand placement is essential for success on this exercise.

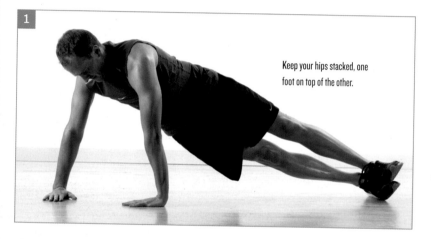

Keep your hips stacked, one foot on top of the other.

Assume a side plank position with your right hand on the floor, fingertips pointing away from the body. Reach across your body and place the left hand on the floor with the fingertips perpendicular to your right hand. Your index fingers should form a 90-degree angle with roughly six inches between the hands.

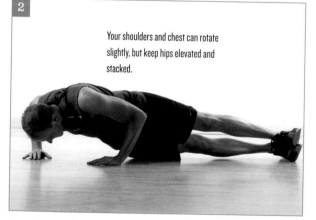

Your shoulders and chest can rotate slightly, but keep hips elevated and stacked.

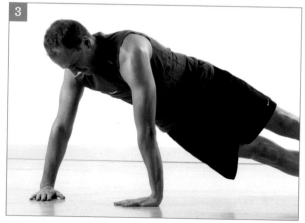

Bend your elbows and lower your chest. Allow the right elbow to bend behind you and the left elbow to tuck to the body, similar to a military or triceps push-up.

Press through the hands, elevating the hips and return to the starting position. Repeat, focusing on correct form over speed.

PLYO PUSH-UP

The push-up is a nearly perfect compound exercise. Adding in an explosive plyometric press and controlled landing will generate incredible upper-body power. Master the traditional and military-style push-ups before attempting this challenging exercise.

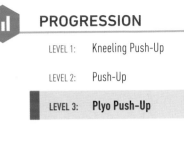
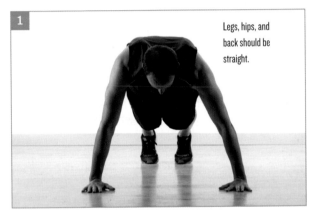

Legs, hips, and back should be straight.

Begin in a traditional push-up position with your core engaged and your body balanced between your toes and hands, forming a straight line from ankles to head.

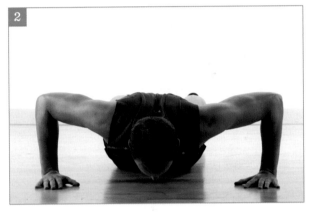

Bring your chest toward the floor until your elbows are bent slightly beyond 90 degrees.

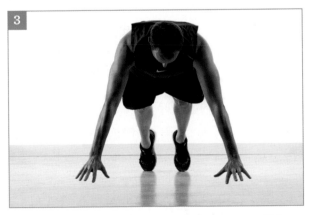

Push up hard enough for your hands to come off the floor. Land with control and repeat.

CHALLENGE

As you gain strength and altitude, challenge yourself by attempting to clap or touch both palms to your chest before landing.

SPHINX

This exercise combines a forearm plank and a push-up to work the chest, triceps, back, core, and hips. It is essential to engage your core throughout this exercise for stability and to protect your lower back.

PROGRESSION

LEVEL 1: Triceps Dip

LEVEL 2: Military Push-Up

LEVEL 3: **Sphinx**

Start in a basic forearm plank position. Your body weight should be evenly balanced between your forearms and toes. Open your hands so that your palms are flat on the floor.

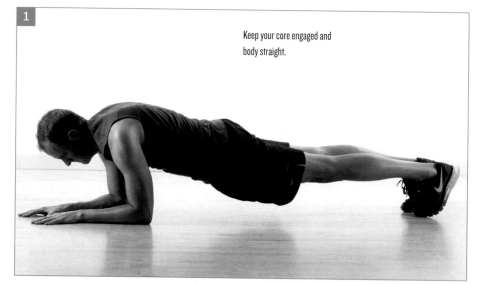

Keep your core engaged and body straight.

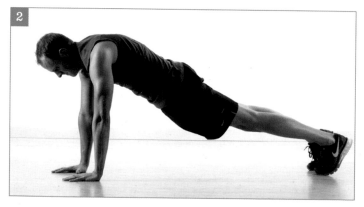

Push through the palms of your hands to elevate your body until arms are straight. Slowly lower back down into a forearm plank and repeat.

TRAINER TIP

If you find it difficult to extend both arms at the same time, build strength by extending one at a time. Follow a pattern of up, up, down, down (right, left, right, left), switching the lead arm with every rep.

REVERSE PUSH-UP

The core-killing reverse push-up is not for the faint of heart. Adding an explosive drive with the legs forces your core to contract in order to slow and stabilize the body. Don't try this exercise if you have not mastered regular push-ups or military push-ups.

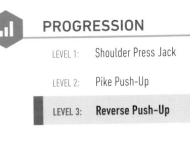
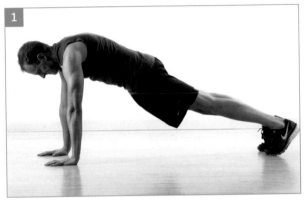

1

Assume a standard push-up position with shoulders over wrists, core engaged, and body forming a straight line from anklebone to shoulders.

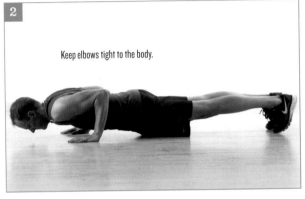

2

Keep elbows tight to the body.

Bend your elbows, lowering until your chest is just above the floor. Keep your core tight and body flat

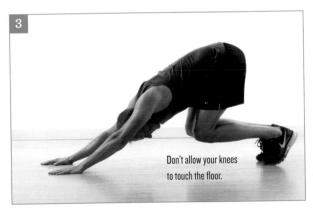

3

Don't allow your knees to touch the floor.

Push back through palms of your hands, bending your legs and pulling your hips back toward your heels. Shift your weight into your heels.

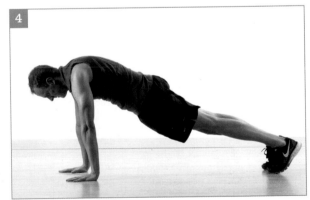

4

Drive through the heels and explode back to a push-up position. Repeat with control, maintaining good form and core engagement throughout.

DRAGON WALK

The dragon walk is a full-body movement that targets your core, chest, abs, triceps, glutes, shoulders, quads, back, and hip flexors. This challenging exercise will leave you breathing fire!

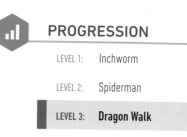

PROGRESSION

LEVEL 1:   Inchworm

LEVEL 2:   Spiderman

LEVEL 3:   **Dragon Walk**

1

Assume a modified military push-up position, with your hands staggered and the right elbow touching the right knee.

2

Press out of the starting position and take a small step forward with your left hand and left foot.

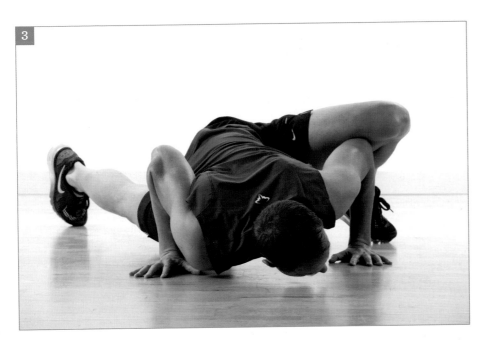

3 Drop back into the staggered military push-up position, this time with the left elbow touching the left knee.

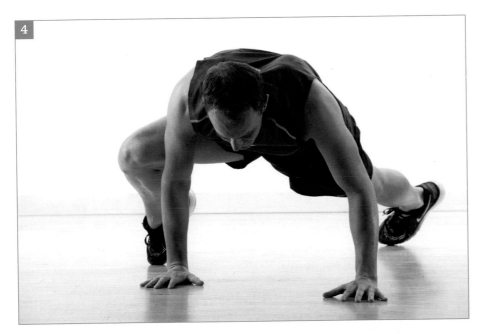

4 Repeat with controlled movement, alternating sides.

PLYO TRIO

If you've mastered all the push-up variations in this book and are ready for a challenge, then take on the plyo trio. By explosively pressing off the floor and landing with a different hand position each time, this trio targets your entire upper body.

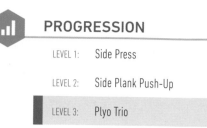

PROGRESSION

LEVEL 1: Side Press

LEVEL 2: Side Plank Push-Up

LEVEL 3: Plyo Trio

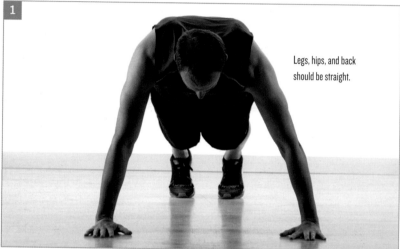

Legs, hips, and back should be straight.

Begin in a traditional push-up position, with your hand just wider than shoulder width apart. Your core should be engaged and your body should form a straight line from ankles to head.

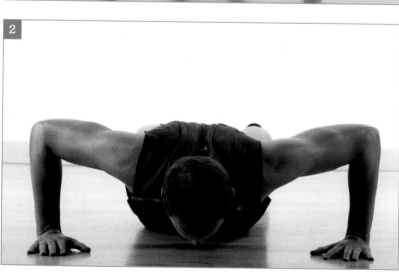

Lower your chest toward the floor, bending your elbows slightly beyond 90 degrees.

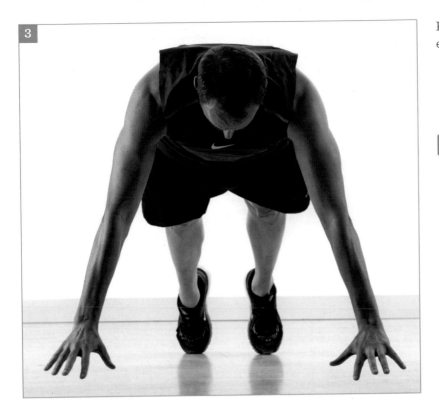

3 Push up through your palms with enough force to lift off the floor.

⚡ **CAUTION**

As you push your body and lift off of the floor, be sure to keep your core engaged. Land with control, using your elbows, wrists, and core to absorb the impact. Landing with straight arms could cause injury. Practice on your knees before tackling the movement from a standard push-up position.

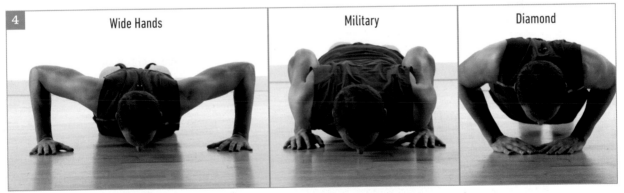

4 | Wide Hands | Military | Diamond

Land with your hands wider than shoulder width apart. Repeat the movement, alternating your hand position each time you land.

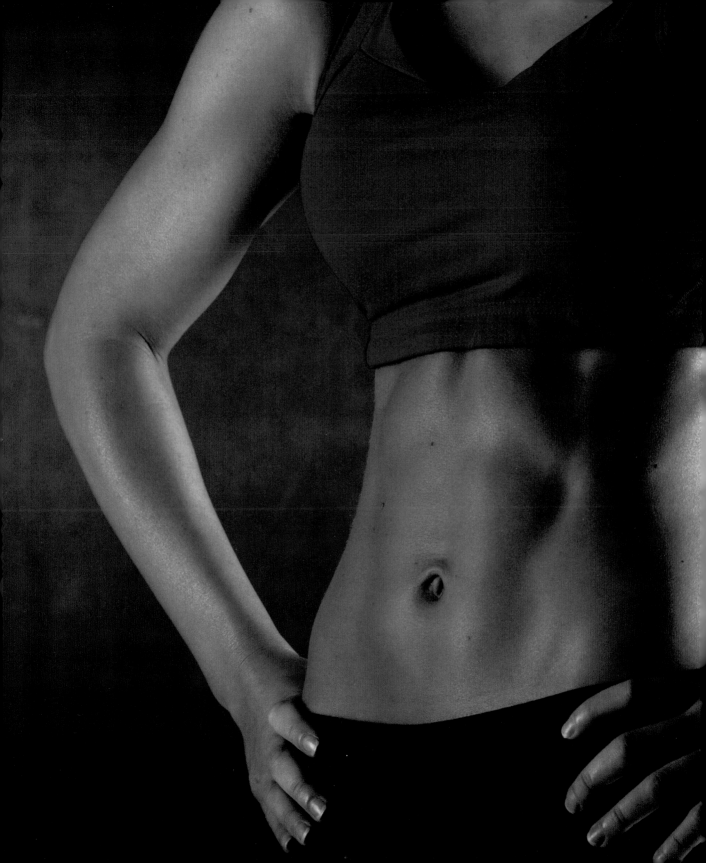

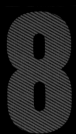
Although almost every exercise in this book works your core as a stabilizer, the exercises in this part specifically target the muscles of your abdomen and lower back to build strength, balance, muscle tone, and definition. The exercises range in difficulty from Level 1 to Level 3. Level 3 exercises are the most challenging, and involve more dynamic movement. Check the level progression guide for each exercise and scale your workout accordingly.

PLANK

This deceptively simple exercise is the secret to rock-hard abs. The plank position engages the transverse abdominals, which aid in stabilization of the spine and pull in the tummy. It helps develop strength in the core, shoulders, and glutes.

PROGRESSION

LEVEL 1:	**Plank**
LEVEL 2:	Diagonal Mountain Climber
LEVEL 3:	1-2 Push

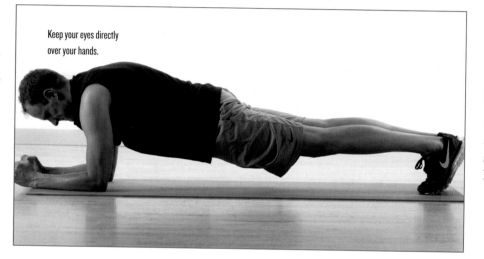

Keep your eyes directly over your hands.

Place your forearms on the floor and extend your legs until your body is balanced between your toes and forearms. Your elbows should be directly beneath your shoulders and your body should form a straight line from head to heels.

CHALLENGE

Try one of these variations to increase the difficulty of your plank.

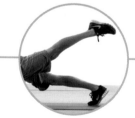

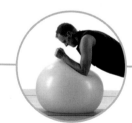

Lift one leg: Lift one leg and extend it upward. Keep your hips square with the ground and resist the urge to rotate.

Lift one arm: Extend one arm straight out in front of you.

Use a stability ball: Rest your forearms on the ball while keeping your toes on the floor. Keep your hips down and engage your core to prevent the ball from rolling.

BICYCLE CRUNCH

PROGRESSION

LEVEL 1:	**Bicycle Crunch**
LEVEL 2:	Double-Cross Reach
LEVEL 3:	Flutter-Up

The bicycle crunch is an excellent exercise for building core strength and toning the thighs. The movement of your legs mimics the motion of riding a bike.

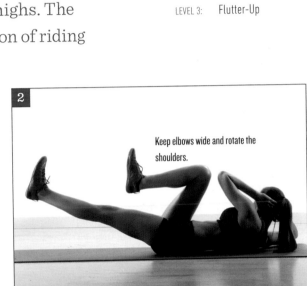

1

Don't pull on your neck.

Lie flat on the floor with your hands behind your head, elbows out wide, and fingers interlocked. Lift your shoulder blades off of the floor by activating the abs.

2

Keep elbows wide and rotate the shoulders.

Elevate your legs until your heels are several inches from the floor. With the left leg extended, bring your right knee toward your chest until it is bent at 90 degrees. Simultaneously rotate your core to pull your left shoulder toward the right knee.

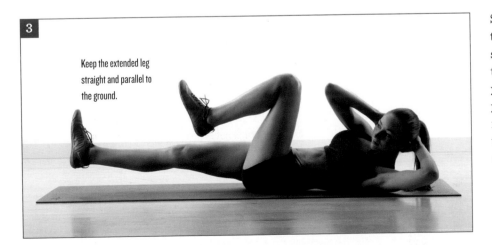

3

Keep the extended leg straight and parallel to the ground.

Switch sides, extending the right leg and simultaneously pulling the left knee toward your chest. Rotate your core and pull your right shoulder toward the left knee. Repeat, alternating sides.

PIKE

The pike, or leg raise, is the one ab exercise I always come back to in the studio. Pikes are a simple yet highly effective way to target your lower abs and hip flexors.

PROGRESSION

LEVEL 1:	**Pike**
LEVEL 2:	V-Up
LEVEL 3:	V-Up Doubles

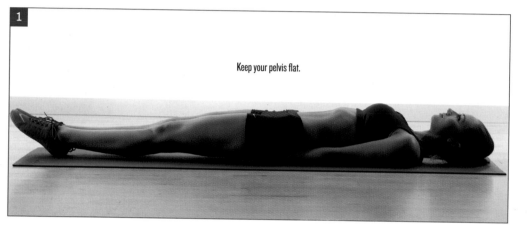

Keep your pelvis flat.

Lie on your back and place your hands under your hips with palms facing down. Keep your legs as straight as possible and squeeze them together.

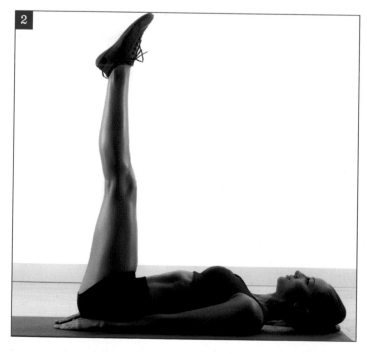

Slowly raise your legs until they are perpendicular to the floor. Hold the contraction at the top for a second and slowly lower your feet to within an inch of the floor.

CAUTION

If your back arches as the legs lower, you are taking your legs too low. The weight and leverage of the legs is too much for your core to control. Adjust the angle of the legs accordingly to keep the work in the abs and hip flexors.

SIDE PLANK

The side plank will tighten and shrink your waistline by working the underlying abdominal muscles (obliques and transverse abs).

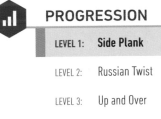

PROGRESSION

LEVEL 1:	**Side Plank**
LEVEL 2:	Russian Twist
LEVEL 3:	Up and Over

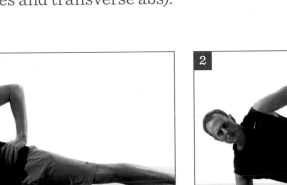

Lie on your side with your legs straight and your forearm on the floor.

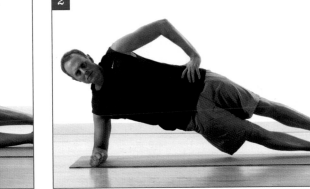

Lift up at the hips, creating a straight line from head to heels. Rest the non-working arm on your hip or behind your head. Hold the position.

CHALLENGE

Add some variety to your workout with these side plank variations.

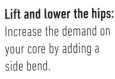

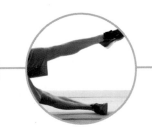

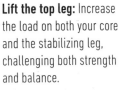

Lift and lower the hips: Increase the demand on your core by adding a side bend.

Lift the arm overhead: Lengthen your body and challenge your stabilizing muscles.

Lift the top leg: Increase the load on both your core and the stabilizing leg, challenging both strength and balance.

CIRCLES

This exercise focuses on the *rectus abdominis,* the internal and external obliques, and the *transverse abdominis.* It's an incredible way to tone, tighten, and strengthen your core.

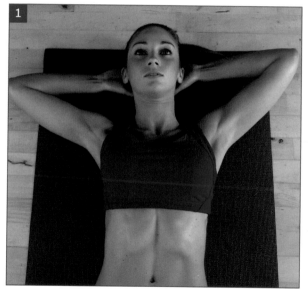

Lie on your back with your legs bent and feet flat on the floor. Place your hands behind your head with elbows out wide. Lift your shoulder blades, engaging the abs.

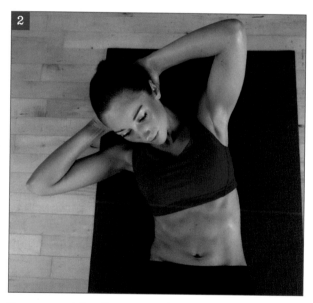

Drop your right elbow toward the right hip and engage the obliques.

CHALLENGE

Once you've mastered the basic circles movement, challenge yourself with these variations.

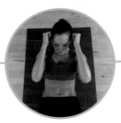

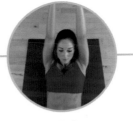

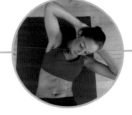

Boxer Circles Bring your guard up and make the circles tighter and faster. Duck and weave!

Rib Cage Isolations Extend the arms overhead and make tight circles, isolating the ribcage and core.

Figure 8 Alternate the direction of your circles. This can be applied to the basic circles or the advanced variations.

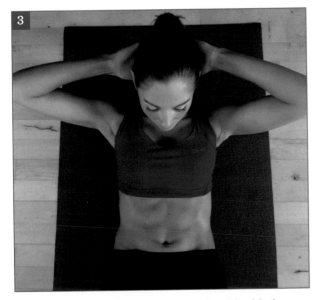

Deepen the crunch by lifting your shoulder blades higher and rotating to the center.

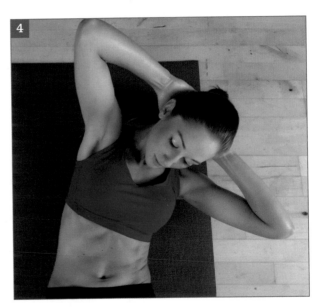

Drop the left elbow toward the left hip and engage the obliques before returning to the starting position.

DIAGONAL MOUNTAIN CLIMBER

Adding a cross-body knee pull to the classic mountain climber adds a dynamic stability challenge. A favorite of my clients in studio, the diagonal mountain climber will take you to the summit.

PROGRESSION

LEVEL 1:   Plank

LEVEL 2:   **Diagonal Mountain Climber**

LEVEL 3:   Flutter-Up

1 Keep your hips down.

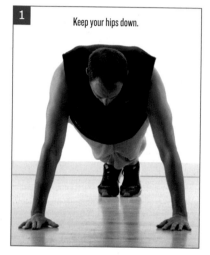

2 Mentally engage your core and squeeze your abs.

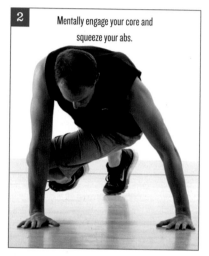

3

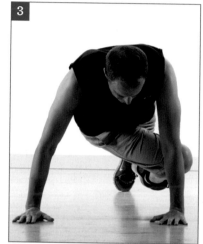

Position your hands on the floor slightly wider than shoulder width apart. Rise up onto your toes and engage the core to form a straight line between your ankles and head.

Pull your left knee forward and across your body to the back of the right elbow. Make sure your knee comes all the way across the body to maximize engagement of the core.

Extend the left leg and simultaneously pull the right knee toward the left elbow. Continue alternating legs, moving as rapidly as possible while maintaining proper form.

CHALLENGE

Try elevating your hands on a small step, bench, or a stability ball to increase the difficulty of this exercise.

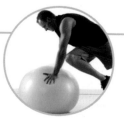

V-UP

The V-up takes its name from the shape your body forms during the exercise. This advanced ab exercise engages the six-pack abdominal muscles, the erector muscles of the spine, and the hip flexors. V-ups require great coordination as well as balance.

PROGRESSION

LEVEL 1: Pike

LEVEL 2: **V-Up**

LEVEL 3: V-Up Doubles

CORE EXERCISES

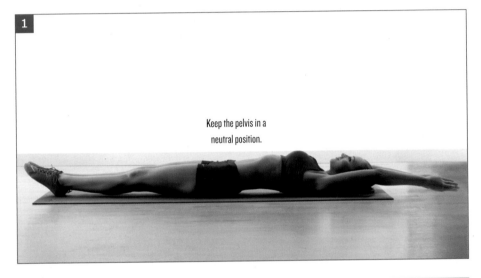

1

Keep the pelvis in a neutral position.

Lie on your back with arms and legs straight. Extend your arms above your head.

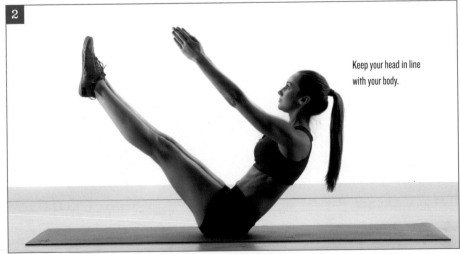

2

Keep your head in line with your body.

In one fluid motion, simultaneously lift your torso and legs. Extend your arms so they are parallel to the legs. Control the body back to the starting position and repeat.

DOUBLE-CROSS REACH

PROGRESSION

LEVEL 1:	Bicycle Crunch
LEVEL 2:	**Double-Cross Reach**
LEVEL 3:	Flutter-Up

The double-cross reach will test your balance and coordination while working your abs, back, thighs, and hip flexors.

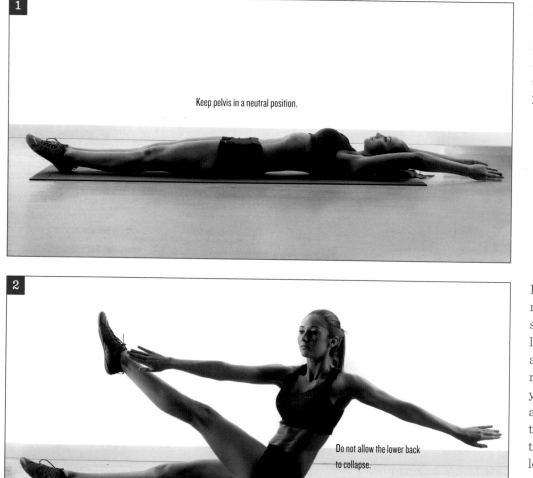

1

Keep pelvis in a neutral position.

Lie on your back with legs straight and arms extended above your head.

2

Do not allow the lower back to collapse.

In one fluid motion, simultaneously lift your torso and legs, reaching with your right hand across the body to touch the toes of your left foot.

CAUTION

This advanced exercise can stress the lower back. If you have lower back pain or injury, substitute the bicycle crunch instead.

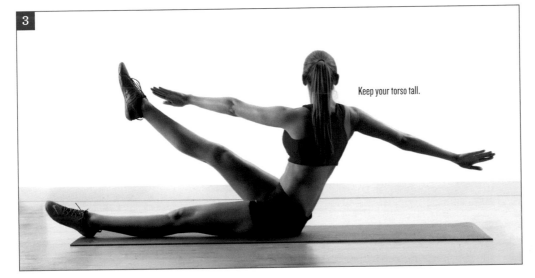

3

Keep your torso tall.

Scissor the legs so that your left hand touches the toes of your right foot.

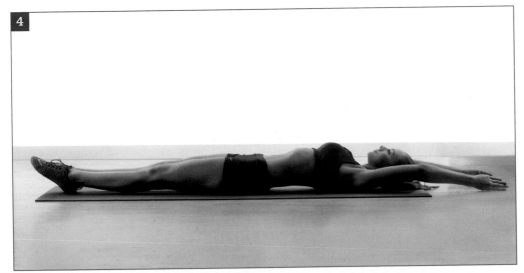

4

Slowly lower back to the starting position and repeat, this time beginning by touching the left hand to the toes of the right foot.

Double-Cross Reach 193

FLUTTER-UP

PROGRESSION

LEVEL 1:   Bicycle Crunch

LEVEL 2:   Double-Cross Reach

LEVEL 3:   **Flutter-Up**

This exercise adds a flutter kick to the V-up, which increases the demand on the stabilizing muscles of the core. The flutter-up is a guaranteed core killer that will get results.

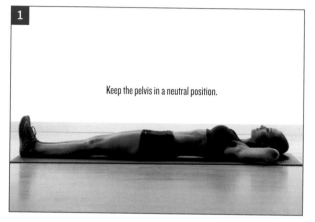

Keep the pelvis in a neutral position.

Lie on your back with arms and legs straight and hands behind your head.

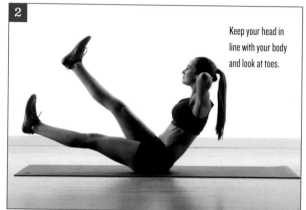

Keep your head in line with your body and look at toes.

Flutter the legs as if treading water while simultaneously lifting the legs and torso until your body forms the shape of a V.

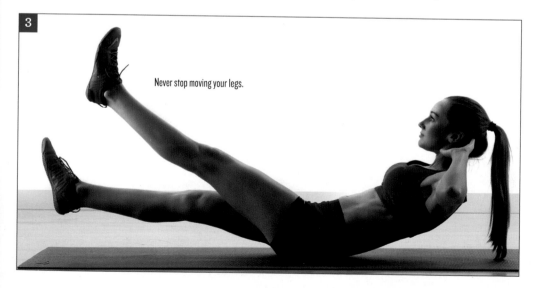

Never stop moving your legs.

Continue to flutter kick the legs as you slowly lower your torso back to the mat.

CORE EXERCISES

IN-AND-OUT ABS

PROGRESSION

LEVEL 1: Plank

LEVEL 2: **In-and-Out Abs**

LEVEL 3: Sprinter Sit-Up

In-and-out abs combines the core work of the classic plank with a dynamic tuck that challenges the thighs and hips and engages stabilizing muscles.

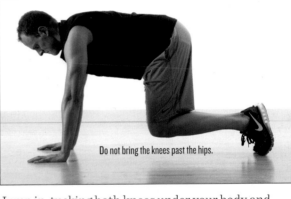

Squeeze the glutes to support your lower back.

Do not bring the knees past the hips.

Begin in a plank position, with hands slightly wider than shoulder width apart. Your body should form a straight line from ankles to head.

Jump in, tucking both knees under your body and landing on your toes with your legs bent at 90 degrees.

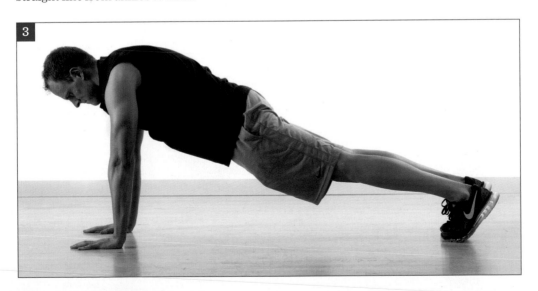

Jump back to the starting position, engaging the core for stability. Repeat.

RUSSIAN TWIST

This classic ab exercise targets the obliques, but your back muscles will also be engaged to stabilize and support your spine.

PROGRESSION

LEVEL 1:   Side Plank

LEVEL 2:   **Russian Twist**

LEVEL 3:   Up and Over

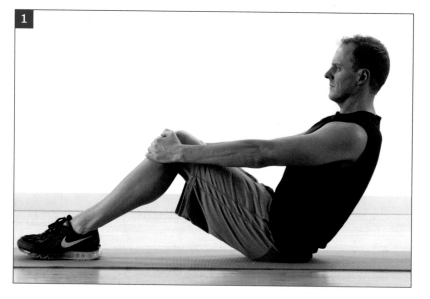

Sit with your knees bent and your heels on the floor. Hold onto your knees and straighten your arms as you lean back without rounding your spine. This is the perfect position for your spine; don't let it curve during the exercise.

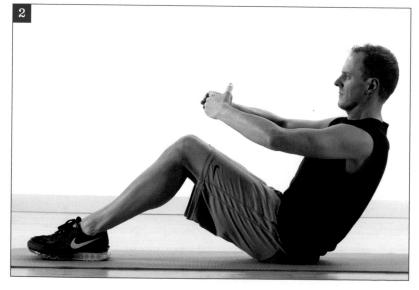

Lift arms from knees and extend in front of rib cage. Arms remain slightly rounded as if holding a beach ball to your chest

CAUTION

Do not do this exercise if you have lower back pain or injury. Substitute the bicycle crunch instead.

CHALLENGE

To increase the difficulty of this exercise, elevate your feet. For an even greater challenge, elevate and extend the legs.

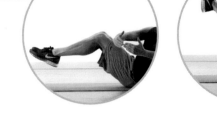

3

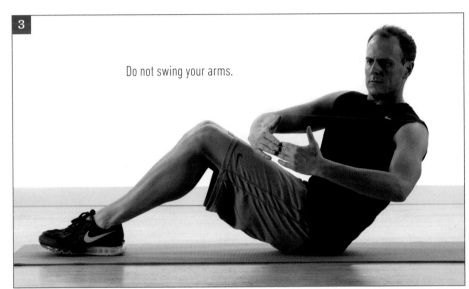

Do not swing your arms.

Pull your belly button to your spine and rotate to the left. This is a small, controlled motion. If you feel pain in your lower back, reduce the amount of twist.

4

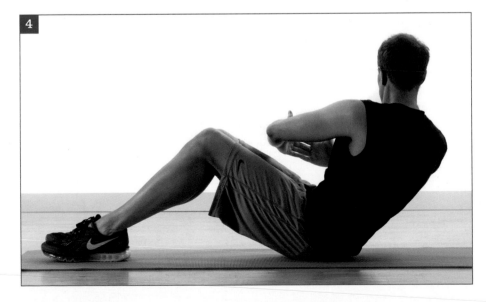

Inhale to center and rotate to the right. Repeat, keeping your abs engaged and spine straight.

V-UP DOUBLES

V-up doubles build on the traditional V-up with an isolation hold of the legs and a second elevation of the torso. This breaks up the exercise, slowing it down and making it harder to use momentum to carry the load. This advanced ab exercise engages the six-pack abdominal muscles, the erector muscles of the spine, and the hip flexors. V-ups require great coordination as well as balance.

PROGRESSION

LEVEL 1: Pike

LEVEL 2: V-Up

LEVEL 3: **V-Up Doubles**

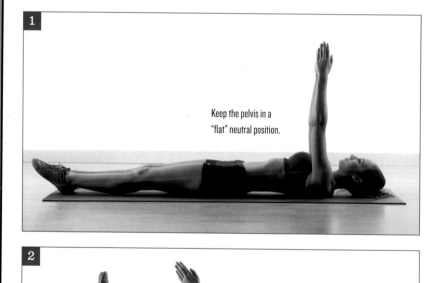

1 Keep the pelvis in a "flat" neutral position.

Lie on your back with arms and legs straight. Extend your arms straight to the ceiling.

2 Keep your head in line with your body.

In one fluid motion, simultaneously lift your torso and legs. Extend your arms so they are parallel to the legs and reach forward to touch your toes.

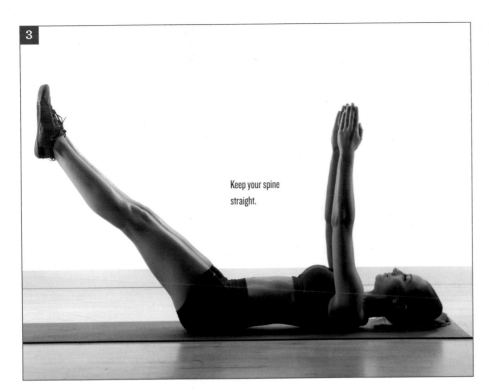

3

Keep your spine straight.

Lower your torso back to the floor in a controlled motion, keeping your legs and arms elevated.

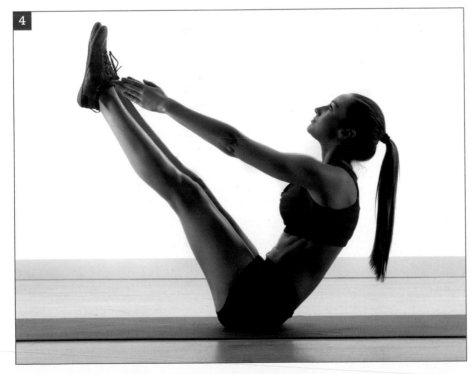

4

Engage your core and lift the torso again in a fluid, controlled motion. Touch your toes. Control the body back to the starting position and repeat.

SPRINTER SIT-UP

PROGRESSION

LEVEL 1: Circles

LEVEL 2: In-and-Out Abs

LEVEL 3: **Sprinter Sit-Up**

This is no ordinary sit-up. The alternating movements of the arms and legs will force your stabilizing core muscles to work, while aggressively driving the knees works the hip flexors.

Lie on your back with your arms at your sides and legs extended.

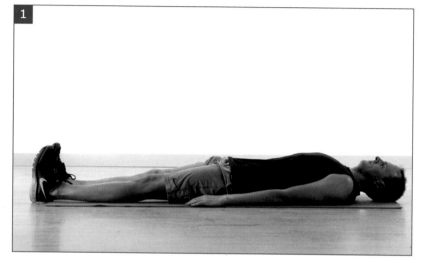

Sit up with an explosive movement, simultaneously bringing the right knee to your chest and swinging the left arm forward, as if running.

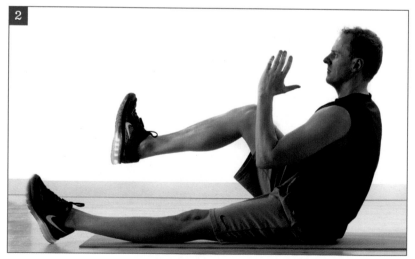

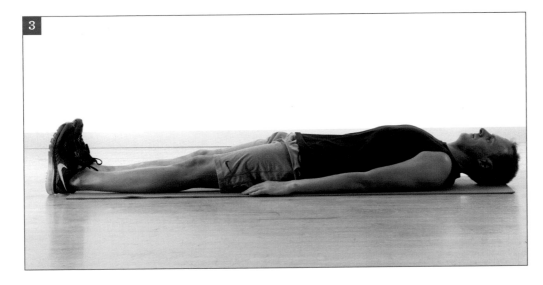

3 Fully extend the right leg and return the left arm to the starting position.

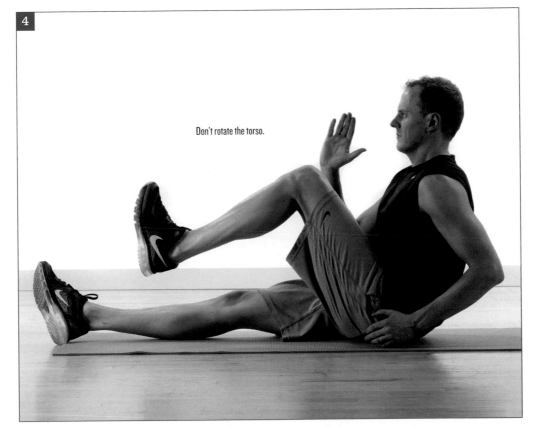

Don't rotate the torso.

4 Sit up again, this time bringing the left knee in to the chest as you swing the right arm forward. Repeat, alternating arm and leg movements, as though sprinting.

UP AND OVER

This balance-oriented ab exercise targets the obliques and hip flexors, but your back muscles will also be engaged to stabilize and support your spine.

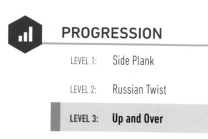

PROGRESSION

LEVEL 1:   Side Plank

LEVEL 2:   Russian Twist

LEVEL 3:   **Up and Over**

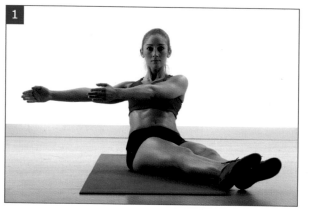

Sit on ground with your legs extended 45 degrees to the left of your torso. Extend your arms in the opposite direction of the legs, 45 degrees to the right of your torso.

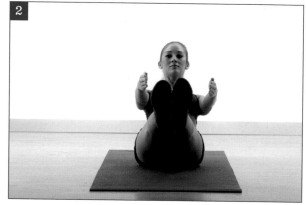

Elevate the feet from the floor and swing them up and over to the right. Simultaneously move your arms in the opposite direction, counter-balancing your body.

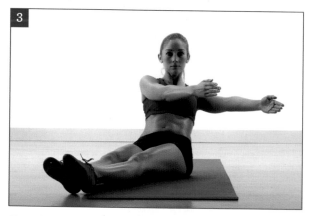

Complete the movement with your feet on the floor, 45 degrees to the right of the torso. Repeat with control, alternating sides.

CHALLENGE

Lean back and lengthen your torso on each swing, keeping your feet up the entire time.

TRAINER TIP

You may find it helpful to stand a yoga brick on its end so you have a physical object to swing the legs up and over.

CORE EXERCISES

1-2 PUSH

The 1-2 push is an intense, full-body move that will elevate your heart rate while working the muscles in your core, arms, and legs. To this day, it is the one exercise I cannot do while simultaneously yelling to motivate my clients. Complete the move as quickly as you can, but remember that form comes first.

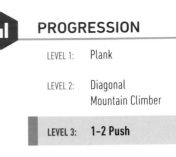
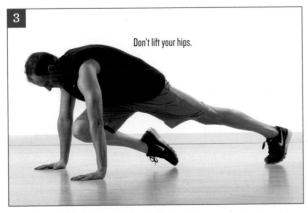

Begin in a push-up position, with hands slightly wider than shoulder width apart. Engage the core.

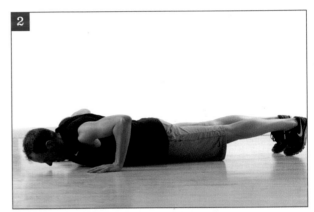

Bend your elbows, bringing the chest toward the floor. When your elbows are bent slightly beyond 90 degrees, push up off the floor and extend the arms.

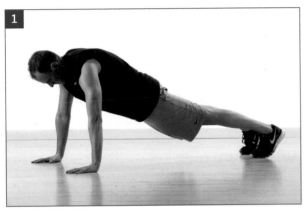

Don't lift your hips.

As arms reach full extension, bring your right knee to your chest.

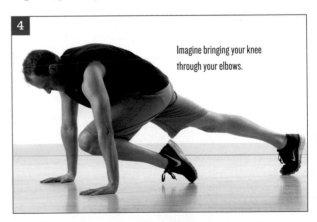

Imagine bringing your knee through your elbows.

Quickly switch legs, bringing the left knee to the chest. Return to starting position and repeat.

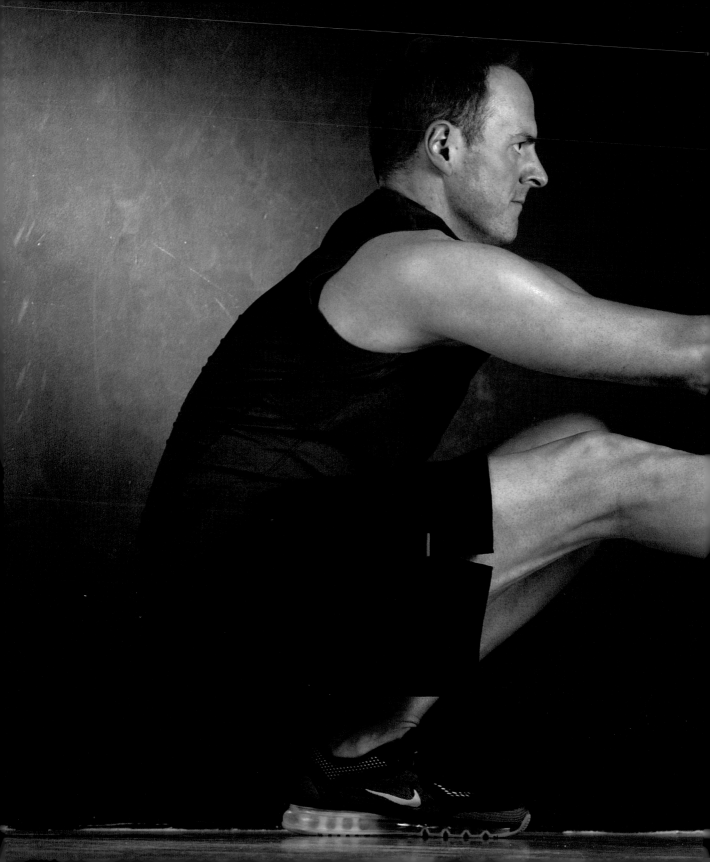

The muscles of the legs are some of the largest in the body, and moving those muscles requires big energy in the form of calories. Nothing fires up your metabolism like squats, lunges, and plyometric (jumping) exercises. The exercises in this part target the legs, including hips and glutes. They are designed to build strength and muscle tone while improving athletic performance. If you find a particular exercise too simple or too challenging, check the exercise progression guide for an alternate exercise that will work the same muscles.

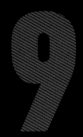

LOWER-BODY
EXERCISES

SQUAT

The body weight squat is a compound, full-body exercise that primarily engages the muscles of the thighs, hips, and butt. It also helps to develop core strength by engaging the lower back and abdominals.

PROGRESSION

LEVEL 1:	**Squat**
LEVEL 2:	Squat Jump
LEVEL 3:	In and Outs

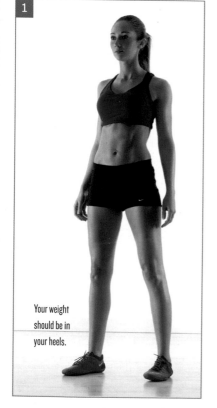

Your weight should be in your heels.

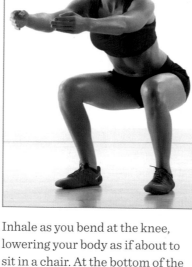

Keep knees over ankles and torso tall.

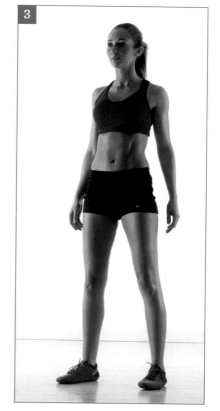

1 Stand tall, with your feet shoulder width apart and toes pointing forward.

2 Inhale as you bend at the knee, lowering your body as if about to sit in a chair. At the bottom of the movement, your knees should be at a 90-degree angle and your thighs parallel to the ground.

3 Exhale as you press through your heels, returning to the starting position. Squeeze your glutes as you stand, tucking your pelvis under and pulling the belly button inward to engage your core.

REVERSE LUNGE

The reverse lunge is a simple, low-impact way to strengthen the quads, hamstrings, glutes, and calves.

PROGRESSION

LEVEL 1:	**Reverse Lunge**
LEVEL 2:	Pedal
LEVEL 3:	Squat Pedal

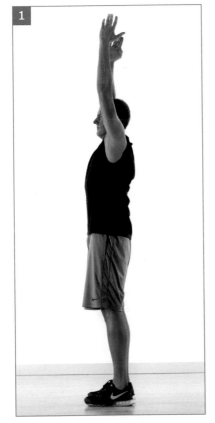

Stand tall with hands overhead.

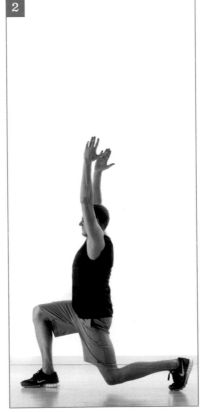

Take a large, controlled step backward with your left foot. Lower your hips so that your right thigh is parallel to the floor and your right knee is directly over your ankle. Your left knee should be bent at 90 degrees, pointing to the floor and directly under your hip.

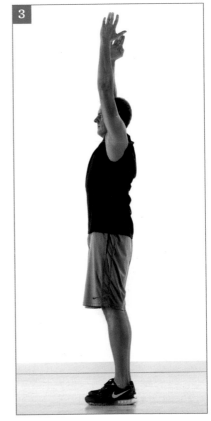

Return to a standing position by pressing through the heel of the right foot and bringing your left foot forward, standing tall to engage the core. Repeat, this time leading with the right leg.

LATERAL LUNGE

Lateral lunges increase dynamic balance, strengthening and toning the glutes, hamstrings, and thighs in the process.

PROGRESSION

LEVEL 1:	**Lateral Lunge**
LEVEL 2:	Lateral Lift
LEVEL 3:	Skater Jump

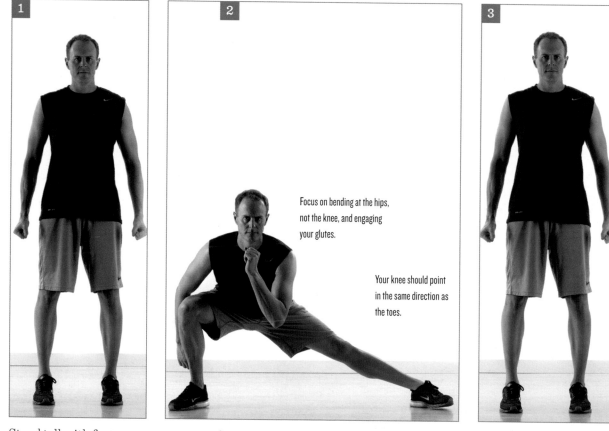

Focus on bending at the hips, not the knee, and engaging your glutes.

Your knee should point in the same direction as the toes.

1 Stand tall with feet shoulder width apart and toes pointing forward.

2 Step out to the side (laterally) away from the body. Remain tall and keep your weight in your heel as you push back your hips, lowering your body until the thigh is parallel to the floor.

3 Push back off of the bent leg, extending hips and knee to return to the starting position.

PELVIC PEEL

The pelvic peel builds strength in the hips, hamstrings, and glutes while simultaneously stretching the quadriceps and hip flexors. Pelvic peels are an excellent exercise if you suffer from pelvic back pain, as they work the muscles that support and stabilize the pelvis.

PROGRESSION

LEVEL 1:	**Pelvic Peel**
LEVEL 2:	Pigeon or Butterfly Peel
LEVEL 3:	Single Leg Peel

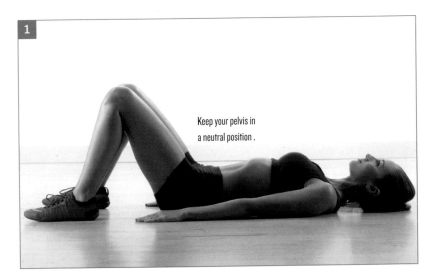

Keep your pelvis in a neutral position .

Lie on your back with your legs bent and your feet flat on the floor. Your arms remain loose by your sides.

TRAINER TIP

The closer you move the heels to your glutes the harder the exercise becomes. For an added stretch, extend your arms overhead and stretch out as long as possible.

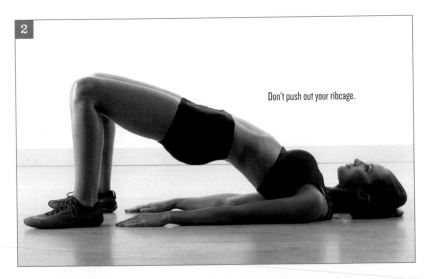

Don't push out your ribcage.

Press evenly through the soles of the feet, squeeze the glutes, and lift the hips until your body forms a straight line from shoulders to knees. Pause at the top of the motion and hold for one to two seconds before lowering back to the floor in a controlled movement.

T-STAND

Lengthen the hamstrings and challenge your balance in this yoga-inspired, functional exercise. While it may seem simple, it will fatigue your hamstrings, glutes, and lower back if done correctly.

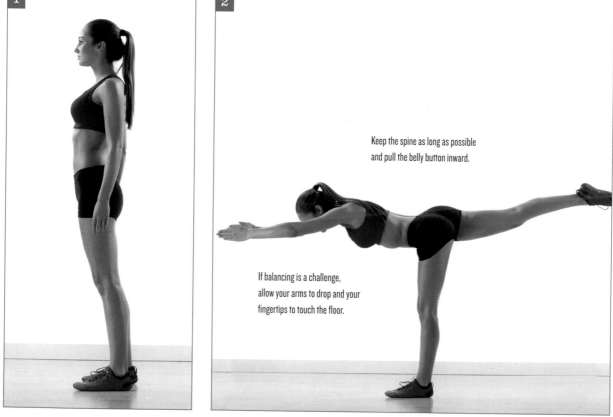

1

2

Keep the spine as long as possible and pull the belly button inward.

If balancing is a challenge, allow your arms to drop and your fingertips to touch the floor.

Stand with feet together and arms at your sides.

Inhale and slowly bend from the hips, lowering the torso and extending the arms. As you fold forward, raise one leg until torso, arms, and leg are parallel to the floor.

Exhale as you lift the torso and lower the leg in one fluid motion. Repeat with the opposite leg.

SQUAT JUMP

A metabolic-boosting super exercise, the squat jump requires focus and coordination. It works all the large muscles of the lower body, including the quads, glutes, and hamstrings.

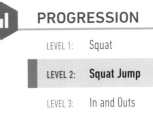

PROGRESSION

LEVEL 1:   Squat

LEVEL 2:   **Squat Jump**

LEVEL 3:   In and Outs

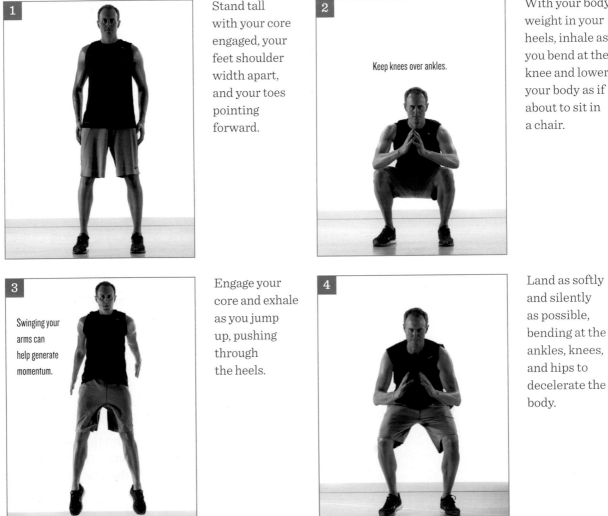

1 Stand tall with your core engaged, your feet shoulder width apart, and your toes pointing forward.

2 Keep knees over ankles.

With your body weight in your heels, inhale as you bend at the knee and lower your body as if about to sit in a chair.

3 Swinging your arms can help generate momentum.

Engage your core and exhale as you jump up, pushing through the heels.

4 Land as softly and silently as possible, bending at the ankles, knees, and hips to decelerate the body.

PEDAL

The pedal, or jump lunge, will quickly get your legs burning and your heart rate skyrocketing. This quad-killing exercise requires balance and coordination. Make sure you're maintaining proper form throughout the movement.

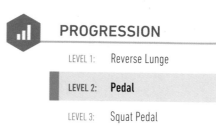

PROGRESSION

LEVEL 1: Reverse Lunge

LEVEL 2: **Pedal**

LEVEL 3: Squat Pedal

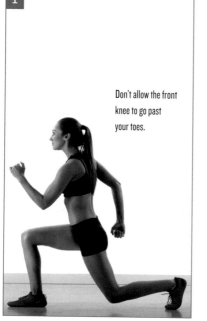

Don't allow the front knee to go past your toes.

Stand with one foot in front of the other. Keep your torso as tall as possible as you bend both legs to sink into a lunge position.

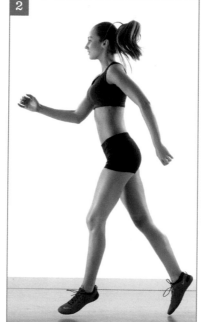

Jump up with enough force to propel both feet from the floor. While in the air, scissor-switch your feet.

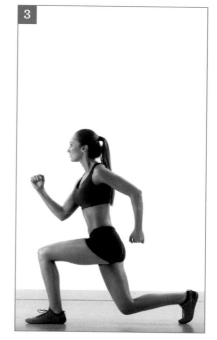

Land in a lunge position with the opposite foot in front. Repeat.

CAUTION

Pay attention to the impact imposed during the landing. Attempt to land as softly as possible so that the force of the deceleration is distributed between the knee, hip, and ankle joints.

SKATER JUMP

This exercise mimics the movement of a speed skater moving across the ice. Skater jumps will strengthen your legs while improving balance and coordination and raise your heart rate in the process.

PROGRESSION

LEVEL 1:   Lateral Lunge

LEVEL 2:   Lateral Lift

LEVEL 3:   **Skater Jump**

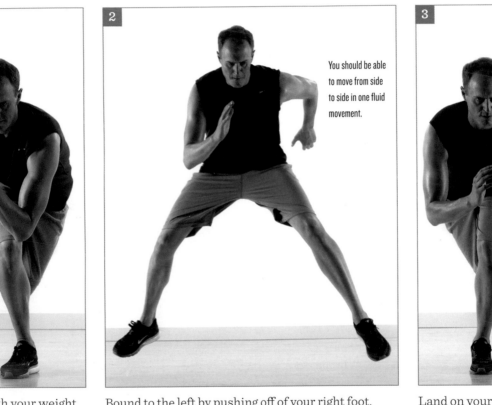

You should be able to move from side to side in one fluid movement.

1 Stand with your weight on your right foot and a soft bend in the knee. Cross your left foot behind your right ankle and lower into a half-squat.

2 Bound to the left by pushing off of your right foot. Swing your arms across your body in the direction of your jump.

3 Land on your left foot and bring the right foot behind your left.

T-STAND KICK

Adding a front kick to the already unstable T-stand takes athleticism and balance. In exchange, it will work the core, quads, hamstrings, glutes, and lower back.

PROGRESSION

LEVEL 1:   T-Stand

LEVEL 2:   **T-Stand Kick**

LEVEL 3:   Log Hop T-Stand

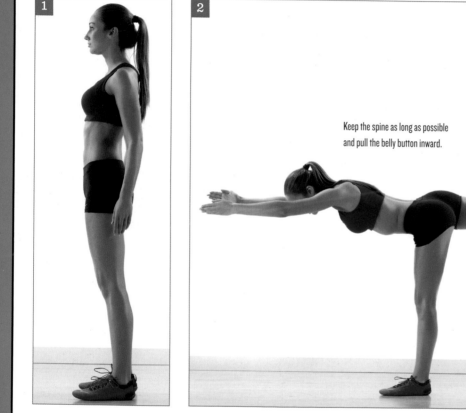

Keep the spine as long as possible and pull the belly button inward.

Stand with feet together and arms at your sides.

Inhale and slowly bend from the hips, lowering the torso and extending arms. As you fold forward, raise one leg until torso, arms, and leg are parallel to the floor.

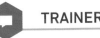

TRAINER TIP

Engage abs for power and balance during kick. Challenge yourself to perform every rep without allowing the kicking leg to touch the floor.

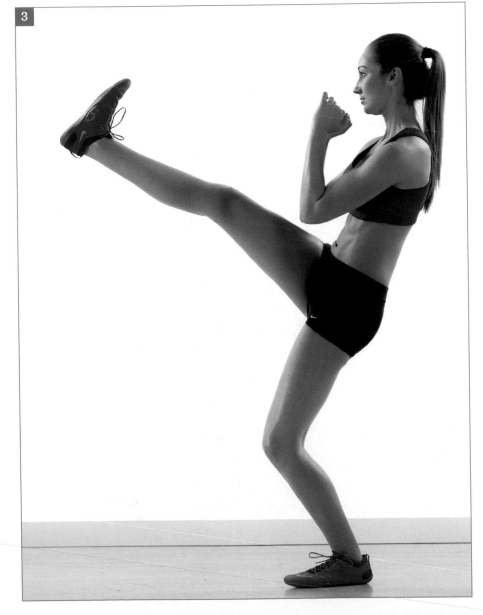

3

Exhale as you lift the torso and bring the extended leg forward, lifting the knee until the thigh is parallel to the floor and kicking the foot up.

PIGEON PEEL

The pelvic peel builds strength in the hips, hamstrings, and glutes. These two variations internally and externally rotate the legs, providing a far greater challenge.

PROGRESSION

LEVEL 1:   Peel

LEVEL 2:   **Pigeon or Butterfly Peel**

LEVEL 3:   Single Leg Peel

Lie on your back with your legs bent and your feet flat on the floor, slightly wider than shoulder width apart. Roll your inner thighs together and squeeze them tight.

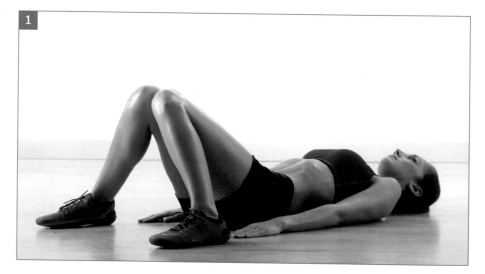

Press evenly through the soles of the feet, squeeze the glutes, and lift the hips until your body forms a straight line from shoulders to knees. Keep your thighs together. Pause and hold for one to two seconds before lowering back to the floor in a controlled movement.

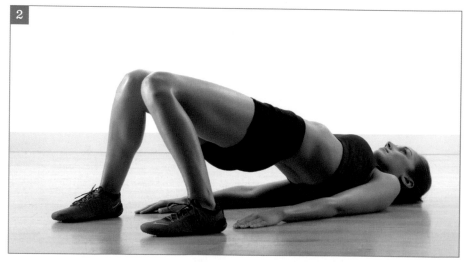

BUTTERFLY PEEL

Lie flat on your back. Bring the soles of your feet together and open your knees as wide as possible.

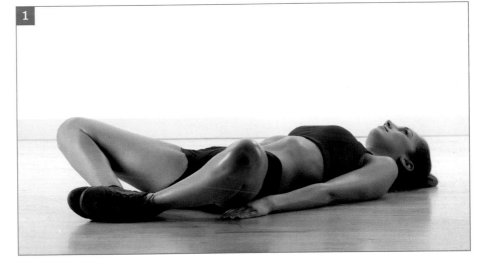

Press evenly through the feet, squeeze the glutes, and lift the hips until your body forms a straight line from shoulders to knees. Do not allow your knees to come together. Pause and hold for one to two seconds before lowering back to the floor in a controlled movement.

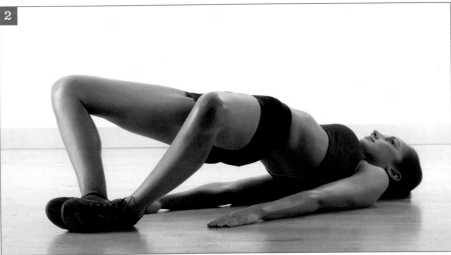

TRAINER TIP

Moving your feet closer to your glutes will increase the challenge of these exercises. Try reaching your arms overhead for an added stretch.

SQUAT PEDAL

The squat pedal combines squat jumps and jumping lunges, creating a powerhouse movement that burns more calories than any other body weight resistance exercise. This metabolic booster simultaneously activates the thighs, hamstrings, glutes, and core. Keep your movements explosive, but maintain proper form.

PROGRESSION

LEVEL 1:   Reverse Lunge

LEVEL 2:   Pedal

LEVEL 3:   **Squat Pedal**

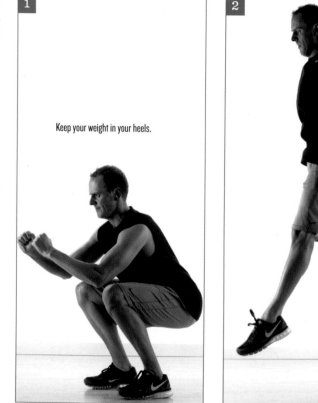

Keep your weight in your heels.

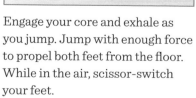

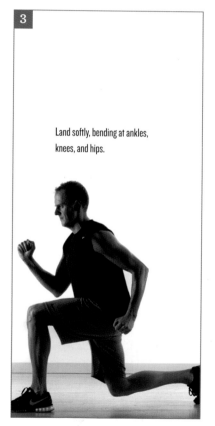

Land softly, bending at ankles, knees, and hips.

1 Stand tall, with your feet shoulder width apart and toes pointing forward. Inhale as you bend at the knee and lower into a squat position.

2 Engage your core and exhale as you jump. Jump with enough force to propel both feet from the floor. While in the air, scissor-switch your feet.

3 Land with the left foot in front. Sink into a lunge position.

TRAINER TIP

If jumping is too strenuous, you can do a combination of squats and reverse lunges.

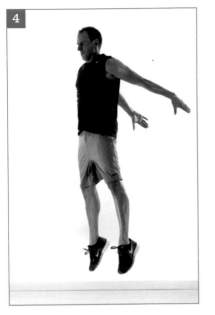

From the lunge position, jump up again with enough force to propel both feet from floor.

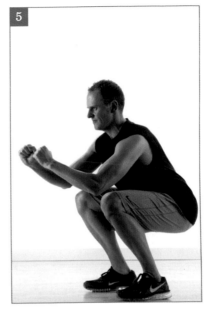

Land back in a squat with feet shoulder width apart.

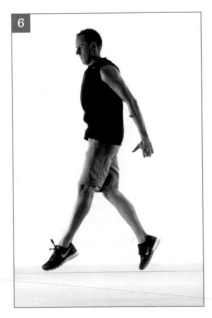

Explode up from the squat position. While in the air, scissor-switch your feet.

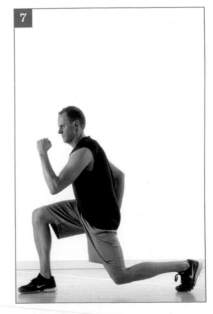

Sink into a lunge position and repeat, alternating squats and lunges.

IN AND OUTS

This plyometric squat engages the thighs, glutes, and hamstrings. It will challenge your balance and coordination, activate the core, and sculpt the lower body.

PROGRESSION

LEVEL 1:   Squat

LEVEL 2:   Squat Jump

LEVEL 3:   **In and Outs**

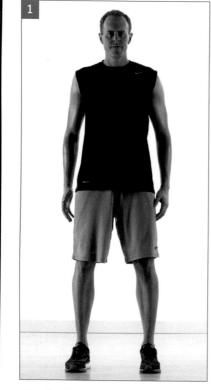

Stand tall, with your feet hip width apart and toes pointing forward.

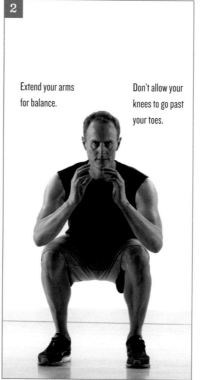

Extend your arms for balance.

Don't allow your knees to go past your toes.

With your weight in your heels, inhale as you bend at the hips and knees, lowering into a squat. Try to bring your thighs parallel to the floor.

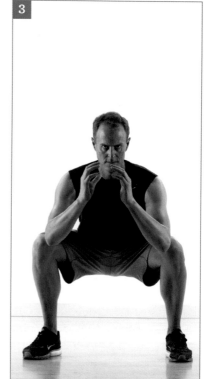

Make a small jump and open your feet laterally, landing with feet slightly wider than shoulder width apart. Repeat, staying as low as possible in your squat position and jumping "in and out."

SINGLE LEG PEEL

PROGRESSION

LEVEL 1: Pelvic Peel

LEVEL 2: Pigeon or Butterfly Peel

LEVEL 3: **Single Leg Peel**

This twist on the pelvic peel increases strength in the hips, hamstrings, and glutes while simultaneously stretching the quadriceps and hip flexors. Elevation of a single leg increases the demand on your core and provides a stability challenge.

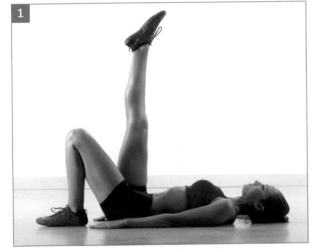

Lie flat on your back. Place one foot on the floor approximately one foot from your glutes and extend the other leg straight to the ceiling (perpendicular to the body). Keep your arms loose by your sides.

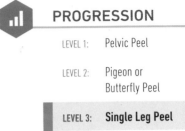

Press evenly through the sole of the foot on the floor, squeeze the glutes, and lift the hips until your body forms a straight line from shoulders to stabilizing knee. Pause and hold for one to two seconds before lowering back to the floor in a controlled motion.

TRAINER TIP

The closer you move the heel to your glutes the harder the exercise becomes. For an added stretch, extend arms overhead and reach as long as possible.

CAUTION

Do not allow your hips to rotate. Keep your pelvis flat and square to the ground throughout the exercise.

LATERAL LIFT

Lateral lifts add dynamic stability to the traditional lateral lunge, forcing you to engage the hip complex and core simultaneously.

PROGRESSION

LEVEL 1: Lateral Lunge

LEVEL 2: **Lateral Lift**

LEVEL 3: Skater Jump

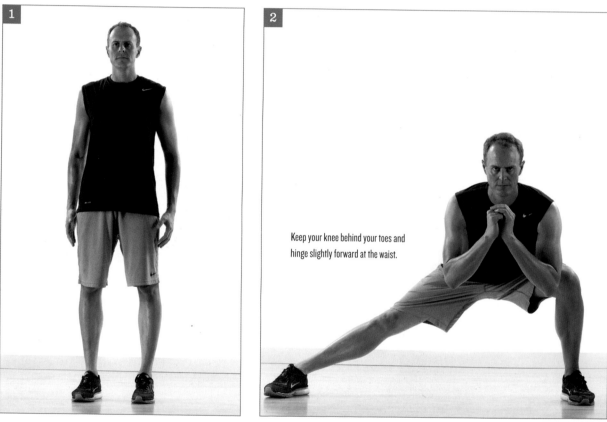

1 Stand with your feet hip width apart, arms straight, and palms facing your legs.

2 Keep your knee behind your toes and hinge slightly forward at the waist.

Step your left leg out to the side and bend your left knee, lowering into a lateral lunge.

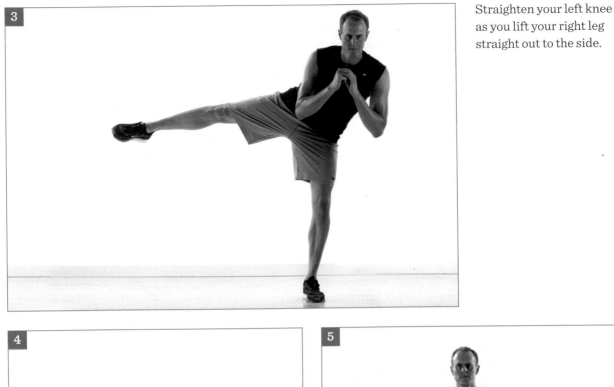

Straighten your left knee as you lift your right leg straight out to the side.

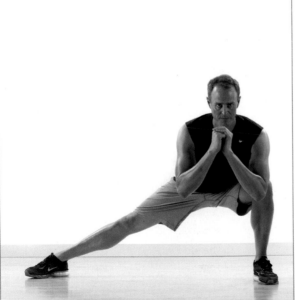

Carefully return to the lateral lunge position.

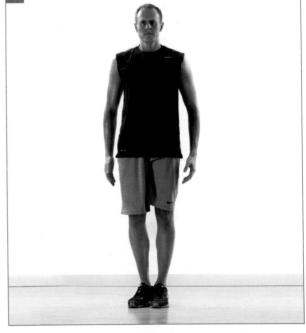

Return to a standing position by pressing through the heel of the left foot and engaging the core, quads, and glutes. Repeat on the opposite side.

LOG HOP T-STAND

PROGRESSION

LEVEL 1:   T-Stand

LEVEL 2:   T-Stand Kick

LEVEL 3:   **Log Hop T-Stand**

Adding an explosive hop to this traditional hamstring, glute, and lower-back exercise will challenge your balance and improve athletic performance. Go slowly until you are comfortable with the instability caused by your lifted leg.

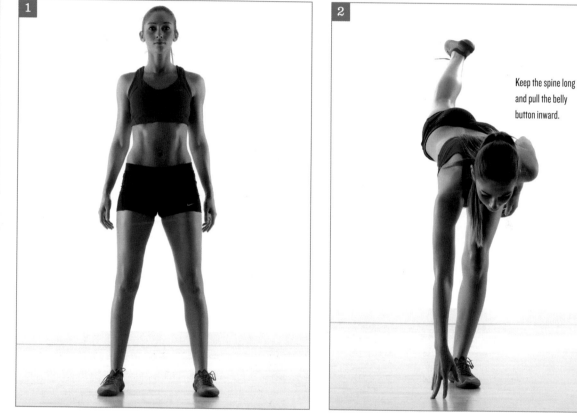

Keep the spine long and pull the belly button inward.

Stand tall with your feet together, arms hanging loosely at your sides.

Inhale and slowly bend from the hips, lowering the torso and extending arms. As you fold forward, raise one leg until your torso, arms, and leg are parallel to the floor.

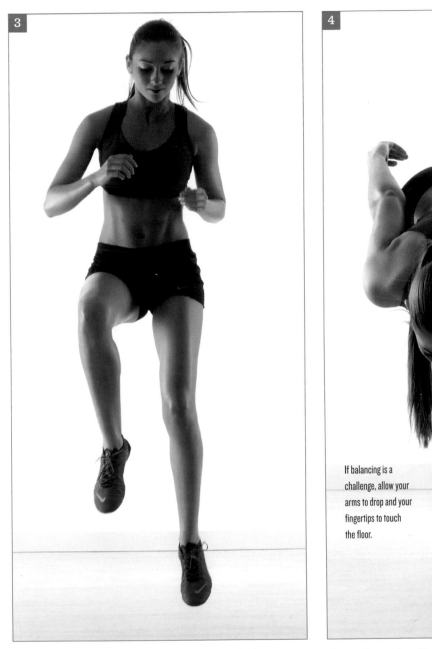

3

4

If balancing is a challenge, allow your arms to drop and your fingertips to touch the floor.

Exhale as you lift the torso and dynamically leap forward, tucking the extended leg to your chest followed immediately by the stabilizing leg, as if hopping over a small log.

Control your landing by engaging the core and absorbing the impact through a triple bend at your ankles, knees, and hips. Lower the torso and raise the opposite leg. Repeat, alternating sides.

INDEX

All photos by Matt Bowen, with exception of the following: p 15, DK Publishing